God's Miracles . . .

Max, the faithful family dog was diagnosed with a brain tumor and given only months to live. God had other plans for Max.

Butch the Cat, lost in the unfamiliar wilds of the Colorado mountains, and rescued by prayer.

The severely abused chow who became "God's little miracle" when his impossible recovery became nothing less than a phenomena.

Serge, the cat who came in from the cold—a loving stray who turned a skeptical couple into firm spiritual believers.

The animal communicator who turned to prayer to aid her dying horse.

The Malaysian energy healer who brings new life to pets.

And . . .

The Baptist Church in Maryland that opens its doors to ailing animals—of all faiths.

Miraculous Pet Recoveries

Inspiring True Stories of Love
and Healing for All
God's Creatures

Les Sussman

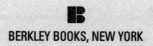

BERKLEY BOOKS, NEW YORK

MIRACULOUS PET RECOVERIES

A Berkley Book / published by arrangement with the author

PRINTING HISTORY
Berkley edition / August 2002

Copyright © 2002 by Les Sussman
Book design by Julie Rogers
Cover design by Judith Murello
Cover photograph by Tim Davis

Visit our website at
www.penguinputnam.com

ISBN: 0-425-18577-X

BERKLEY®
Berkley Books are published by The Berkley Publishing Group,
a division of Penguin Putnam Inc.,
375 Hudson Street, New York, New York 10014.
BERKLEY and the "B" design
are trademarks belonging to Penguin Putnam Inc.

PRINTED IN THE UNITED STATES OF AMERICA

10 9 8 7 6 5 4 3 2 1

To my grandfather Joseph Sobel, who would never harm a fly, and to my mother, Chaya Fryda, who taught me that all of nature is filled with God's presence.

And God made the beast of the earth
after his kind,
and cattle after their kind,
and every thing that creepeth
upon the earth after his kind;
and God saw that it was good.

GENESIS 1:25

. CONTENTS .

▪ FOREWORD ▪

IN December of 1999, my standard poodle, Sandy, was suffering from what a veterinarian diagnosed as a herniated cervical disk. She gave me medication for him, but warned that he needed to be kept quiet because too much movement could cause the disk to impinge upon the spinal cord, resulting in paralysis.

Sandy and I share a very close bond, and I was very worried about him. Although I belong to the prayer line at my parish, I felt awkward asking the other members to pray for my dog. Most pet owners are familiar with the odd looks we sometimes get from people who are not animal lovers when we talk about our pets.

One night, I was praying for Sandy when I suddenly remembered something that happened several weeks before Sandy fell ill. While I was on-line reading the "Prayer Intention" message boards on a Christian website, my attention had been captured by the subject line of one of the postings. It said: "Please pray for my dog." The message was from a woman named Marlowe who was requesting prayer for her sick dog, Chauncy. I e-mailed Marlowe and told her I would be praying for her dog and she wrote back to thank me. It now occurred to me that I should write Marlowe and ask her to pray for *my* dog. I went to my computer and dashed off an e-mail, and within minutes Marlowe replied, writing that she would add Sandy to her prayers.

It was then that an idea began to take form in my mind: *Wouldn't it be wonderful if there were a prayer line just for animals? Then people with ailing or lost pets would not have to feel hesitant about asking for prayer for their beloved animal companions.*

Although such prayer lines probably existed, I was new to the Internet and did not know of any. So I decided to start my own. I e-mailed Marlowe again and told her my idea and asked if she was interested in being part of the prayer chain. She readily agreed, and the Pet Prayer Line was born. I then started to recruit other members and developed a website. We now have people on our prayer chain from all over the United States and overseas, and we handle numerous prayer requests every day. The prayer line is nondenominational and open to people of all faiths.

If you visit the Pet Prayer Line website and see our on-line prayer list, you will notice that there is a "People List" along with an "Animal List." This is because shortly after the Pet Prayer Line started, I began to get prayer requests for humans in need. I firmly believe that no one needing prayer should ever be refused, and so I simply added a "People" section to our prayer list. We are all creatures of God and are all in need of His healing touch.

Since the inception of the Pet Prayer Line, I have

had the privilege of seeing many sick animals restored to health and lost animals reunited with their human families.

Sometimes a physical healing is not in God's plan, but even then the power of prayer brings a peaceful passing for the beloved animal companion, and strength and courage to those who mourn this passing. Those who request prayer also benefit from the overwhelming love and compassion of the wonderful people who make up our prayer chain. Countless times they have rallied to the aid of a worried or bereaved pet owner, offering words of comfort, encouragement, and sometimes advice. The Pet Prayer Line, as well as this book, would not have become a reality had it not been for the cooperation of these people, who truly reflect the love and goodness of God in their prayers, words, and actions.

During Sandy's illness, I had a chance to experience for myself the power of prayer in the healing of an animal. One night, a day or two after Sandy had been to the vet and I had been warned about keeping him quiet, I saw Sandy struggling to get up off the floor where he'd been napping.

It was time for him to go out before bedtime, but although he struggled, he couldn't get himself into a standing position. In fact, it seemed that he couldn't move the lower half of his body at all. My heart fell to my feet and I thought, *This is it—he's paralyzed.* I didn't want to force him to get up, for fear of hurting him further. I didn't know what else to do except pray.

I decided to pray over him as my church's prayer group prays over people who are in need of healing. I sat on the floor next to Sandy and I began to pass my hands, palm down, over his body an inch or two above his fur, shaking my hands out after every pass.

As I did this, I prayed and visualized white healing light flowing from God through my hands, and I willed this light into Sandy to heal him. After a few minutes of this, I sat down in a chair and prayed some more. I had just about finished when I saw Sandy trying to get up again. This time he pulled himself up completely and walked over to the back door! You can imagine my joy and relief as I poured out my thanks to God and (carefully) hugged Sandy.

From that point on, Sandy, who is now thirteen years old, started to improve, and thank God, he has had no further trouble with his cervical discs. Would Sandy have been able to get up without my prayers? Possibly. Did the medication have a part in his healing? Of course. But I believe that my sincere and fervent prayer played a significant role in the recovery process.

It is overwhelming to see the increasing number of people struggling to grow spiritually in a world that gives them little in the way of inner joy, serenity, or fulfillment. Our lives are troubled, rushed, and frustrated. Our souls are hungry for the gift of true peace, and we derive hope from hearing about other people's experiences of God in their lives.

This book helps to answer that need, and I feel greatly privileged to have some part in it. In the pages ahead, you will read about the prayers that were answered in the form of miraculous healings of animals.

Each testimonial will give you a feeling of hope and inspire you to try for yourself the wondrous power of prayer. You will feel the joy these people felt when God answered their prayers by healing their pets.

If you read with an open mind and heart, God will touch your life through this book as surely as He has touched theirs. If you take the time to lift your heart in prayer, you will find an unending source of strength and hope.

Sit quietly for a few minutes every day to fill your mind with God's light, and you will see that miracles are not just for others but for *you* as well. Small miracles and big ones—they happen all the time to those who trust in God.

Gloria J. Pinsker, founder, Pet Prayer Line

∙ AUTHOR'S NOTE ∙

ANIMALS have always been an important part of my life. Ever since I was a kid they've been scooting about me in one form or another; cats, dogs, birds—even a reptile or two which my parents weren't too fond of, but I was.

Over the years I've always sensed that these innocent creatures are specially blessed. But it wasn't until I began researching the stories for this book that I began to realize exactly how extensive these blessings are.

After listening to all these amazing and moving testimonies from pet owners across the country whose pets had often been written off as hopeless cases by veterinarians, and then had been given back the gift of health through prayer and other spiritual means, I'm now more convinced than ever that a higher source is looking after our four-pawed and feathered friends.

It makes perfect sense to me that the universe would seek to protect creatures who bring so much joy and comfort into our lives. I am also convinced that prayer is a powerful tool for healing, as the inspiring true stories in this book help to demonstrate.

If you have a pet who is ailing, and your veterinarian seems to have given up hope of its recovery, it is my sincere hope that you will pick up this book and read a story or two. I am certain these testimonies will help not only boost your spirits, but also bring a smile to your face.

Many of these pet owners were also given bad news about their beloved pets, but with faith and prayer the results turned out to be exactly the opposite. The Creator seems to have a soft spot in His or Her heart for our non-human friends.

Finally, I want to thank everyone who shared their stories with me. I know that it can be painful recalling a period of time when a pet was critically ill. I also realize that speaking publicly about such things as a miracle sometimes makes people feel a bit uncomfortable.

I also would like to express my special appreciation to those people I interviewed who, despite a busy lifestyle, volunteer their time to protect and save animals— working with rescue groups or in shelters, hosting websites, and doing whatever else they can to assist our furry friends. You are really wonderful folks and I hope this book in some way pays homage to all your efforts.

The most important point this book makes, and the real reason I am delighted to have written it, is to remind all of us in this scientific age never to give up hope when the chips are down. Miracles can happen. All you need do is believe. . . .

. ACKNOWLEDGMENTS .

I'M indebted to many people for making this book possible. Special thanks to Gloria Pinsker—known as "Rose" on the Internet—the founder of the remarkable Pet Prayer Line. Without her help, there would be no book.

Much appreciation also to Adrien Amadeo, an extremely gifted healer who heads up the Internet's Healapet Network. Her efforts also contributed greatly to the making of this book.

I also want to give special thanks to Carolyn C. Collie, business manager of *The Christian Science Journal,* for her assistance, and to Meredith Puryear at the Association for Research and Enlightenment (A.R.E.) in Virginia Beach, Virginia.

Much thanks also to The Seeing Eye, Inc.; Guide Dogs for the Blind; Bonney and Michael over at the Best Friends Animal Sanctuary in Kanub, Utah, and all the people connected with Dal Savers. Thank you also to "Captain Hook," someone I've never met but who linked me to Eileen Smith and her remarkable story about the resurrection of her dead cat.

I want to thank Edita for putting up with me during those hectic moments when I stressed out while writing this book. Much credit is also due my new agent, Marshall Klein, who loves penguins and was disappointed there was not one miraculous penguin story in this book. Maybe next time, Marshall!

Also much thanks to Denise Silvestro, my editor at Berkley Books, who believed in this book and reported back that members of her editorial board had tears in their eyes when they first read the proposal.

Last but not least, let me squeeze in some much-deserved thanks to longtime friends like Sally Bordwell, Alan Grossman, Claire Gerus, Judith Myers, Karyn Feiden, Andrea Shaw, Patricia A. Leone, and everyone over at New York City's Sanctuary Restaurant, where all spiritually-inclined animal lovers should dine regularly.

1 . A Gift from God

EILEEN Smith, a registered nurse for more than thirty years, says she will never forget the morning three months ago when she awoke to find her six-year-old tabby, Spencer, lying seemingly dead beside her. Nor will the Nashville, Tennessee, resident ever forget the miracle which she says she witnessed some moments later, when Eileen believes her fervent prayers to God to save her beloved pet's life were answered.

It was such an extraordinary event in her life that Eileen says ever since that day she has been reluctant to talk about what happened for fear of being ridiculed. Since that miracle unfolded, she adds, she has only shared her astonishing story with two close friends.

But now Eileen says she is prepared to talk about what happened because she cannot keep the story of a miracle of this magnitude bottled up inside her any longer.

"I received a very special gift that day," she fervently proclaims. "It was the gift of life for an animal that is extremely precious to me. This cat was given back to me by God."

. . .

If anyone is qualified to offer an informed opinion about whether an animal is alive or dead, Eileen Smith certainly is. Although she is not a veterinarian, the former New Yorker has worked as a registered nurse for more than three decades, and over the years has operated both an animal rescue group and shelter. Her familiarity with animals, in fact, dates back to when she was a young girl growing up on Long Island. "My family had a small piece of property, and we had cats and dogs, rabbits, pigeons—the whole nine yards. And I used to bring home homeless animals all the time," she admits.

As she grew older, Eileen recalls always being surrounded by pets. Even today, her home is crowded with rescued cats and dogs. "I have eight or nine cats and a couple of dogs running around my house," she says. "They're all strays that I've picked up since I've moved here. They're my family. I just love being around animals because they give so much back."

Eileen and her ex-husband operated an animal rescue program on Long Island. "It was called the Homeless Animal Rescue Team," she says. "Then we moved the program to Maine, where we converted an old barn into an animal shelter. We used to neuter strays and adopt them out." Eileen recalls that many of those abandoned animals required medical treatment. "I would use my medical background to care for these animals at the shelter," she explains. "I would do IVs, blood drawing, minor surgery, and all sorts of things.

I've seen plenty of dead animals in my time."

Eileen relocated to Nashville to care for her ailing sister. She got a job working for the state's department of corrections, where she tends to the health needs of death-row inmates at Nashville's Riverbend Maximum Security Prison.

The job, she quickly notes, is not as depressing as many people might believe it to be. In fact, she often finds her work inspiring. "I was brought up Catholic— but not very religiously—and this kind of experience renews your faith in God," she explains. "I've personally seen how religion makes a significant difference in some of these prisoners' lives, and religion becomes a more important part of your own life when you see how it works and the effect it has on other people."

But it was not her prison nursing experience which had the greatest spiritual impact upon her, she says. Rather, it was a cat named Spencer, whom she has owned since her days living back east.

"His mother was a stray who I had taken in," she relates. "This was about 1995, and our rescue was picking up stray cats in the neighborhood all the time. These cats were running free and looking very thin and sickly."

After giving birth to her latest litter, the mother cat died. Spencer was one of three kittens born in that last litter, and it was a difficult birth.

"He was born with a damaged cerebellum. He couldn't walk properly—he was spastic. He resembled someone with cerebral palsy and fell over continually."

After five months of care, Eileen says that Spencer was finally able to stand up and manage by himself, although to this day he still walks with a jerky motion.

"He probably should have been euthanized because he was so much trouble, but he was doing so well that I just left him alone and took care of him. He was a feisty little thing—and he still is. He still has a little trouble walking, but aside from that he's led a relatively healthful life."

The grayish-black kitten bonded to her from the beginning, Eileen recalls, and she returned Spencer's love and affection. "I became like a mother to this cat," she laughingly states.

After her divorce, Spencer accompanied Eileen on her journey westward, and became her unseparable companion. "When I sleep he lies by my side and he kind of lies in a spooning fashion cuddled up against me," she relates. "When he comes to me he starts purring so loud, I can feel it."

Three months ago, Eileen awoke one morning and immediately sensed that something was wrong. "He wasn't purring. And when I kinda pulled him toward me, he was a little cool. He just didn't feel right. Usually he has all these jerky movements."

When she took a closer look at Spencer, Eileen remembers feeling shocked. "As a nurse, I know reality. I know dead," she states unequivocally. "I've worked with dying patients and animals long enough. And believe me, this animal was dead. I know what I saw."

Eileen pauses, her voice cracking with emotion as she relives that horrifying moment. "There was nothing about him that suggested to me he was alive. There was no muscle tone, his eyes were lifeless, and his head was dangling at an angle, like a rag doll. It was awful. My heart broke," she attests. "This was one more terrible thing that had happened to me recently.

I had undergone a divorce, my sister was seriously ill—and now this. It was overwhelming. I was very upset."

At that grief-stricken moment, Eileen says she did what comes naturally to her—she turned to prayer. "I remember I said these four words that were addressed to God: 'Please, God, not now!' My whole life was falling apart and this little baby was so precious to me. He was the one thing that made me smile. And then I picked him up and prayed some more."

Eileen remembers cradling Spencer in her arms and rocking him like a child. "I was thinking, 'Maybe I'm wrong. Maybe it's not true that he's dead.' I was hoping against hope that he was still alive. But nothing had changed. There was no life to him at all."

Again Eileen pauses in the telling of her story, fighting back tears. "I just can't express how I felt at that moment. It's so painful for me to think about that right now." She composes herself and continues.

"I was sitting there looking at Spencer, and about twenty minutes later, I see his tail twitching. I just couldn't believe it. I absolutely knew as a nurse that he was dead. And then, little by little, he started to have these small tremors. But his head was still listlessly hanging to the side."

Again she pauses. "You know, I've only told two people this story because I knew that nobody would believe me. But it's all true. Over a period of about five minutes, there were these little twitches."

Then came the most amazing moment of all, one which Eileen talks about with a sense of awe in her voice. "All of a sudden he snapped to! It was like, 'Whoa, here I am.' I just can't explain it. His head just snapped up. And he started purring again, just like he always did. There was a glow coming from him and he started nipping at my face."

There were more tears, she recalls, but these were tears of joy. "I was so grateful—so overjoyed," she exclaims. "I just knew that my prayers had been answered. So many painful things had happened to me, but now I was given a gift. This cat was given back to me by God."

2 . The Lost-and-Found Kitten

MELODY Pugh, a Bremerton, Washington, pet detective, says that in the past three years she has located more than nine hundred lost and stolen animals. She credits her high success rate not to any special investigative skills but, rather, to the help of a very special "spiritual partner" who assists her with every case.

Melody says she discovered her "spiritual partner" when her own kitten, Norman, was lost for more than three months in April of 1995. Without God's help, she asserts, Norman would still be a name on the missing pets list.

Her search for Norman is more than just a lost-and-found pet story. It is also the account of a woman who for many years felt lost herself, and then, in the midst of her ordeal, found what God intended for her to do with the rest of her life.

. . .

The first time I spoke to Melody on the phone, the upbeat forty-five-year-old pet detective was a bit out of breath. She apologetically explained that she has just come back from a wearisome afternoon tramping through a nearby swamp in search of a missing dog.

Tramping through swamps, looking in all sorts of hidden places for lost and stolen animals, is all part of the job for this former police officer, who admits she never dreamed that one day she would be tracking down missing pets instead of contending with two-legged mischief makers.

Melody, who was raised a Seventh-Day Adventist, recalls that religion always played an important part in her family life, but that its influence waned a bit when she was old enough to leave home.

For many years, Melody always felt as if "something were missing. I was searching for God, or something in my life, that would help make a difference. I always wanted to make some kind of meaningful contribution to the world."

That search led Melody to a series of law enforcement jobs after she dropped out of college. "I majored in go-find-a-job," she quips, "and I was attracted to law enforcement."

One of those jobs was with the Portland Oregon Police Department. It was a position she held for eight years. Melody left the department in 1988 to join her husband, Gary, a former army engineer, who had found work in Washington State.

"This uprooted me again, and once more I found myself trying to figure out where my place in the world was supposed to be," she says. Not certain what to do next, Melody accepted a position doing security work at a nearby U.S. government–operated shipyard.

For the entire two years that she worked at the navy base, Melody says that always, somewhere in the back of her mind, there was a nagging feeling that something important was still missing in her life. "I gave it my all, but I knew I was destined to be doing something else. I just didn't know what."

It was on a spring day in 1995 that Melody unknowingly took the first steps toward finding what she had long been searching for. That day, she and Gary decided to find a new cat to help them get over the recent death of a beloved pet.

"We were heartbroken and were looking for a kitty that resembled our old cat, who was a Manx with a short tail," she recalls. "It wasn't easy to find.

"One day a neighbor who lives across the street came over and told us that one of her children's cats had a litter, and that I would find exactly the kind of cat we were looking for."

The neighbor was not exaggerating. Both she and Gary immediately fell in love with the week-old blue-eyed kitty, whom Melody laughingly describes as the "ugliest one of the litter." Melody says she purposely selected the ugly duckling "because from my own experience those are the ones that over the years usually turn out to be the most loving and have the most beautiful personalities."

She was not wrong. The gray, silver, and brown-colored kitten proved to be as lovable as Melody thought he would be. "Norman was a really good kitty and was beginning to flourish," she exclaims. "He got along well with the other seven cats we have."

A few days later, Melody took the kitten to the veterinarian for his shots. She remembers that it was a beautiful April morning—not a day she ever expected misfortune to befall her.

"I did something that day that I didn't do with any of my cats." She sighs regretfully. "I should have put Norman into a carrier, but for some reason I decided not to.

"I arrived at the vet's office and parked in a lot behind his office. When I opened the car door, some noise scared Norman and he suddenly bolted from the car right into traffic."

Melody says she will never forget what followed. With her heart pounding wildly, virtually frozen with fear, she watched helplessly as Norman dashed through speeding traffic, somehow, miraculously, avoiding being struck by a car.

Moments later, she, too, found herself running through heavy traffic in pursuit of the runaway kitten. "I just couldn't let him die," she declares. "I had to catch him.

"How neither of us was hit by a car I'll never know," she exclaims. "I didn't even hear the squeal of tires because my eyes were directly on Norman—all my senses were directed toward him.

"I ran and ran and ran, and Norman made it across the street and down to a corner and then turned the corner. I got down to that corner as fast as I could, but he wasn't anywhere to be seen. I stayed there and searched that area until five-thirty the next morning."

Exhausted, Melody returned home to get some sleep. Little did she know that her search for the runaway kitten would take ninety-five days and literally change her life.

"From that moment on, every waking hour of the day—except when I needed to go home and eat or sleep—was spent in my search for Norman," she relates. "I even quit my job. Then I spent all my time trying to figure out every way I could find him.

"I called all the local rescue organizations, humane societies, and local veterinarians. Although each place I called was very supportive, they gave me no idea of how to look for him.

"Then I got a call from a guy by the name of David. He said he was a volunteer with one of the rescue services—the Consolidated Lost Pet Line—which is in a town not far from me. He had heard all about my search for Norman. He made me a great lost pet flyer, and I made copies of it. I laminated them and placed them on telephone poles and put them in the windows of any business that would allow me to put them up."

Melody remembers returning home one night after handing out and posting more than two hundred flyers. The light on her answering machine was blinking, and the machine was filled with messages from people who had seen her flyers.

"At first only six calls came in about possible sightings of Norman," she recalls. "Toward the end of the search, there were hundreds. I had taken a total of 646 calls in a ninety-five-day period and posted more than two thousand flyers."

Despite her extraordinary effort, Melody was still not close to finding her missing kitten. "I always seemed to be a step behind him," she says. "Ohhh, how I wanted him home safe in the worst way. My heart was broken and every day continued to be a 'looking for Norman' day."

As she continued her search, Melody heard from more and more people with lost or stolen pets of their own. "People would call and start telling me about their own missing pets," she relates. "Before I knew it, I found myself searching for other lost animals—and finding them—while I was looking for Norman."

During this period, Melody also found herself doing something else differently—relying more upon God for help in finding Norman. Melody says that she began praying a lot, something she had not done much of since her childhood.

"I knew that Norman wasn't just going to walk through the kitty door of my house and show up," she asserts. "So I began pleading with God, talking to Him."

There were doubts, however, she concedes. "I felt that I wasn't doing enough for Him to have my prayers answered. I felt that my prayers were insufficient and that I needed to do more to help God—that I wasn't going about things in the right way. Otherwise, I would have Norman home already."

Melody decided to step up her search efforts. Each day she personally visited a different area where people thought they had seen her missing kitty. "I started introducing myself to people in those areas and telling them my story. I lost twenty-eight pounds walking around looking for Norman." She laughs.

There was a morning when Melody was driving home from the local shelter where she checked in each day, when an event occurred which would forever change her life.

"I remember that I pulled over to the side of the road and I let loose with everything—all the frustration—that had been wrapped up inside of me all these months," she relates. "I just screamed out Norman's name. I screamed, 'Norman, where are you?' at the top of my voice. If anybody had heard me, they would have thought I was crazy.

"Then I began crying. It was the first time I really let it out—not like the regular weepy crying and feeling sorry for myself I had done over the past weeks. I realized that this moment was going to be the make-or-break point for me. I was either going to continue my search or quit."

Melody then began to pray in earnest, and experienced what she describes as an unusual reaction.

"It was as if some voice was speaking to me," she relates. "It was telling me that from this moment on, all my tears needed to be set aside and that I must remain positive about what I was doing.

"I just knew those words were not something I would have come up with—that they were from a separate source. I felt that I was hearing God speak to me and offering me encouragement. That He was finally responding to my prayers. And from that moment on, no matter how many hours I had been out searching for Norman, and no matter how few hours of sleep I got, I always had energy that kept me going. I had an almost certain feeling that I would find Norman."

This God-given encouragement, she adds, arrived at just the right time, because Gary and other members of her family had given up hope of ever finding Norman and were telling Melody to do the same.

"When I told them I would not stop looking for Norman, they seemed a bit surprised, but they offered to continue to help," she recalls. "So the search went on.

In the meantime, I was getting more and more calls from people who wanted me to help them find their own missing pets."

Melody laughingly recollects that during those weeks she spent searching for Norman, she was able to find twenty-seven lost pets and return them to their owners. "I was overjoyed for these people," she declares. "And I didn't let it get me down that I was finding everyone's missing pet but my own. I just knew there was a reason for me still not finding Norman, and that I would eventually be guided to him. I felt refreshed and filled by God's spirit."

She does, however, recall one moment of doubt. "I received a phone call one evening from a local couple who wanted to thank me for helping them to find their missing kitten. I was overjoyed for them, but it was a moment when I felt very low about not finding my own cat yet. So after I hung up the phone, I sat down at the computer and began writing a letter to God.

"I wrote, 'Please bring Norman into the *light of day* so that the kitty angels can bring him home to us.' Then I turned the computer off and visualized the letter being taken to heaven for God to read it. I must say I had never done anything like this before, but right now it seemed as though it was the thing for me to do."

Early the next morning, Melody was awakened by a ringing telephone. "On the other end of the line was a local newspaper carrier, Angie, who my husband and I call Angel. Angie told me that she was delivering her newspapers when she saw one of the flyers I had put up the night before. She remembered seeing a kitten which fit Norman's description, and she and her partner had returned to the area where Norman had been sighted. When they sported the kitten again, they must have spooked it, and it dashed under a house. Her partner had stayed by the hole the cat disappeared into while she went to phone me."

Then Angie made a remark which so startled Melody that she nearly dropped the phone. "She told me that when she was searching for a pay phone to call me, she had uttered a prayer. I asked her what the prayer was, and Angie said that she had prayed, 'Lord, if this is the poor lost kitty needing to be found, please bring him into the *light of day* so that I may see him.'"

It was the exact phrase Melody had used in her letter to God. "When she said that to me, I started running through the house, grabbing my keys and things. I knew immediately that this was the real thing—that it was Norman she had spotted. Gary saw tears streaming down my face and just knew what it must be. He hurried along with me."

Melody says it took her less than five minutes to get going. Believing that time was essential, she ran stoplights and did not slow down at any stop signs in her haste to reach Norman. When she and Gary arrived at the location, Angie and her partner were there waiting for them.

"My husband approached the hole under the house and called Norman's name," she recalls. "Norman let out the biggest kitty cry, one that could be heard all the way to heaven. I just stood in the road and wept.

"Moments later Norman was on his way home with us. He was pretty sedate and his legs didn't work very well for him. He was very weak but *very* happy to be found and going home."

Reflecting back upon that ordeal, Melody declares

that she no longer questions what she should be doing with her life. She is content and satisfied with her work as a full-time pet detective.

Nor does she have any doubts about the presence of God in her life. "I absolutely believe that I am divinely guided in my work," she declares with conviction in her voice.

"I also know that this is exactly the kind of work God wants me to do. He loves animals as much as He loves human beings, and I've become one of His helpers, to help keep them safe."

Since those days, Melody has also become a firm believer in angels. "Without angels," she declares, "I'm positive Norman would never have been found. God and the angels led my way to Norman.

"Without prayer, without God, and without angels, I know in my heart that I would never have found one single lost or stolen pet—let alone the more than nine hundred I've located over the last three years."

3 . A Cow, a Prayer, and a Healing

AT age eighty-four, Laura Briscoe-Powers has had many years to think about a remarkable summer day more than three decades ago when she experienced the instantaneous healing of a dying cow.

What she describes as nothing less than a miracle took place in the small town of Squires, Missouri, where she and her late husband, Chester, once operated a three hundred-acre dairy farm.

When her favorite Jersey cow, Cutie, seemed despondent after the loss of her calf and the local veterinarian could not help the cow, which was growing weaker each day, Laura, a devout Christian Scientist, turned to prayer to help the ailing animal. The retired welder and dairy farmer believes her prayers saved Cutie's life. She points to this miraculous recovery as proof of one of the teachings of her faith, that "under God there are no problems."

Laura further adds that the story of Cutie's healing clearly demonstrates that God is available to help any-

one—animal and human alike—and all it takes is
prayer and faith to move the Creator into action.

■   ■   ■

Although her name was Cutie, Chester called the Jersey cow every other name in the book, Laura laughingly relates. "My husband used to have all kinds of
bad names for her because she used to wiggle every
time he tried to milk her." She chuckles. "He was never
able to milk her quickly, and she never gave a lot of
milk."

Laura nonetheless always had a special affection for
the "small, brown-colored Jersey who was the cutest
little cow in the herd. She was always one of my fa-
vorites, and I always kind of felt sorry for her when
she made my husband mad."

Laura admits that her heart has always gone out to
animals. "All my years growing up, we usually had
dogs and cats around our house," she recalls. "I just
love animals."

Another constant presence in her life was religion.
"My father was a Methodist and my mother was a
Christian Scientist. We were raised religiously, and I
especially loved Christian Science—over the years I've
gotten so much help from it."

During her life, Laura worked a series of odd jobs,
including a stint as a shipyard welder during World
War II.

"When the war ended we decided to look for a place
to permanently settle down. By that time we had a
couple of kids. So my husband made a little trip to the
Ozarks to look around. He liked it there and said we
could buy land at a cheap cost. So we bought the dairy

farm and spent the next twenty-five years trying to pay it off," she says laughingly.

"It wasn't a big dairy farm—about thirty-five cows at the most—and we barely made a living—but we made it! And best of all, we worked together, which was nice."

One of her chores, she recalls, was to check each night to make certain that all the cows had returned home from pasture. "One evening a cow was missing—it was Cutie—and my husband and I were very concerned. The next morning we found her—she was in trouble calving."

Although the veterinarian arrived quickly, Laura recalls that it was too late to save the calf. "It was a difficult situation," she recalls. "Not only did the calf die, but afterward something was wrong with Cutie—we couldn't get her up on her feet no matter how much we tried."

Laura will never be certain whether it was heartbreak or some other reason, but she remembers being told by the veterinarian that he had no idea of how to get the despondent cow back on her feet.

"There was nothing physically wrong with Cutie, but we worried that she might be dying," Laura relates. "For two days and two nights the cow would not get up on its feet. She wouldn't eat or anything, and she was growing weaker. I prayed steadily for her throughout those two days."

When Cutie's condition failed to improve, Laura says she stepped up her efforts and "I tried to pray more earnestly. I loved this cow so much, my heart just went out to her. I prayed to understand that animals, too, are spiritual creatures and part of God's creation."

Laura remembers one day sitting in the field with Cutie and holding the cow's head while she prayed. "Chester and I tried time after time to help her up on her feet, but we couldn't get her up."

Early one morning—three days after Cutie still refused to budge—Laura rode out to the pasture on the back of a tractor driven by her husband. Once more they were on their way to check on the cow's condition and to see if they could get Cutie back on her feet.

"I remember asking myself, 'Am I going to continue praying for this cow?' The answer that came into my head as I jumped off the tractor was 'Yes, I will, because I know that Christian Science heals.' "

Laura says what happened next remains in her mind like a photograph, frozen in time. "I walked over to Cutie, and the other cows were all standing around and staring at her. She was lying there, and I was shocked at the condition she was in.

"My husband said, 'Laura, she's dead.' I thought, 'Well, if she is, I'll be satisfied because I know she died without suffering.' Then my husband saw her wiggle an ear. 'No, she's still alive,' he said. That made me think that I was going to keep praying.

"So I just touched her with my foot and I said, 'Cutie, you are a real problem.' Then, just like a flash, these words came to me—they were as loud as if someone were speaking to me. The words were 'Under God there are no problems.' "

Laura avows that she doesn't believe in "special" miracles, explaining that according to the tenets of her faith, "Christ is constantly among us and is *always* working miracles—it's just that many of us fail to be aware of it." Still, what happened next was a moving experience which she has never forgotten.

"Just when I heard those words—'under God there are no problems'—Cutie's eyes got bright and she was up in a flash. We had a tub of water with us for her to drink, but she just got up and went over to be with the other cows. She didn't even stop for a drink of water."

Laura remembers standing there very still and quiet. "Something happened that morning—words were spoken that even my husband hadn't heard," she says. "When I tried to tell him about it, he just kind of changed the subject. He wasn't a Christian Scientist, so I don't know what he thought. I even doubt that my children believed it when I told them, but what happened that day is all true," she says earnestly.

Nowadays, reflecting back on that special summer morning, Laura says it not only confirmed all the beliefs she has long held about Christian Science, but made her a better Christian Scientist.

"This was the first instantaneous healing I had ever witnessed," she attests, "and now I *truly* understood that under God there are no problems. It made me a real believer in my religion."

4 . A Schnauzer Returns from Death's Door

ROSE Stearns, a nurse for more than thirty years, and her husband, Jay, a physician, have seen their share of sickness and death during their long medical careers.

So when the New Bedford, Massachusetts, couple brought their beloved schnauzer, Princess, bleeding profusely from the mouth and rectum, to the animal hospital, they had little hope of their dog's chances for survival.

But as the Stearns family was soon to learn, miracles do happen and prayer is often the conducting rod.

Today, Rose is eager to share the story of Princess's recovery with anyone who is coping with an ill or seriously injured pet. She is convinced that there is always a chance of survival if one believes in God.

"Open your heart and pray to God," she urges. "He will do what you ask."

■ ■ ■

Rose Stearns says she will always fondly remember that day in 1983 when she and Jay decided to bring home a new dog. One of their neighbor's schnauzers recently had a litter, so the couple decided to have a look.

"Princess actually wasn't the breed we wanted to buy—she was a little gray schnauzer puppy," Rose recalls. "But when we got there, she just wouldn't leave us alone. We fell in love with her.

"That dog loved us as much as we loved her," she continues. "She tried to please us all the time. In fact, if we told her she was eating something bad and to stop, she would actually spit it out."

Things went along fine between Princess and her new owners until, three years later, just as the schnauzer was celebrating her third birthday, tragedy struck. Rose remembers that the day had been proceeding normally enough, with Jay taking Princess out, as usual, for her late-afternoon walk along the beach.

"She loved going outdoors with him. We live on an ocean bluff, and as she did every other day, Princess bounded down the forty-two steps that went from our house to the ocean. It was rocky along the shore and she loved to play and run along those rocks."

It was early evening and Rose was preparing dinner, waiting for Jay and Princess to return home. When they did, Princess did not look well.

"Jay told me that Princess had suddenly disappeared. He went looking for her, and finally found her about a half mile down the beach. When he found her, she just didn't seem right. She was walking slowly, and when they got back here, Princess couldn't get up the stairs easily. She started staggering and weaving, as if she were drunk."

The sight of her beloved pet in such a disoriented condition upset Rose, but she didn't make much of it. "I carried her into the house and figured that she had exerted herself more than usual. My husband had to see patients that evening, so he left and I fed Princess."

Rose hoped the food would help to revive the out-of-sorts schnauzer, but it didn't. "She was usually ravenous all the time, but this time she didn't touch her food," she relates. "Then she disappeared somewhere in the house. I called her, but she didn't respond. I looked everywhere and I still couldn't find her."

That's when Rose became very concerned. "I suddenly had this bad feeling that something was terribly wrong," she recalls. "I've had a lot of experience with pets, and I knew that when an animal is dying, it usually hides. I was frantic."

Rose's worst fears were soon confirmed. "I finally found Princess in the downstairs den under the couch, and she was whimpering." She shakes her head at that vivid memory. "I pulled her out and—my God!— blood was flowing both from her mouth and rectum. She was also in shock."

Dashing to the phone, Rose called her veterinarian and filled him in on the situation. Next she called Jay, who canceled his appointments and quickly returned home. Meanwhile, Rose began utilizing some of her nursing skills.

"I wrapped Princess up in blankets to keep her warm," she says. "I knew she was in shock, but I still had no idea what had happened to her."

With their eleven-year-old daughter, Jennifer, in

tow, the family left for Pilgrim Animal Hospital, where Dr. Robert Boswell was waiting for his patient.

"Dr. Boswell took one look at Princess and said she was definitely in shock," Rose relates. "He said he wasn't sure he could save her because the bleeding was so bad. He had trouble starting an IV because her veins had collapsed.

"Jay and I are both medical people and we realized that Princess was at death's door. The only real question left in my mind was what had caused all this internal bleeding and how could we stop it."

When the doctor finally managed to get an IV into Princess's leg, he told the Stearns that he would stay with Princess all night. He added that he "didn't think Princess was going to make it."

Leaving the animal hospital at about eight P.M., Rose remembers feeling emotionally drained. "I cried all the way home," she recalls. But despite her grief, another feeling settled over her—an optimistic one.

"I don't know what it was, but I just had this sense that she wasn't going to leave us yet," Rose recollects. "Was it God speaking to me? I'm just not sure."

Hearing God's voice would hardly have surprised her at all. "I grew up in a religious family that always believed God's help was always nearby. When I was a youngster, we all went to church each Sunday and I went to Catholic school. As a young girl, I even considered becoming a nun."

When the Stearnses returned home from the animal hospital, the family immediately began praying for Princess's recovery. "We all gathered in the house and talked about what had happened. We prayed, and then we prayed some more."

It was then agreed that each family member would take turns praying for the seriously injured dog throughout the night. "Then I called my in-laws, who are very religious, and they prayed for Princess as well."

There was one more matter to be taken care of, Rose recalls. "We wanted to solve the mystery of what had happened to Princess earlier that evening."

Armed with a flashlight, she and Jay followed the route that the schnauzer had taken on its walk along the beach. Then they found what they were looking for!

"There it was—a half-eaten crab, right where Princess had been playing." Now Rose and her husband understood what had happened. Princess had obviously eaten the crab and the shells had torn her stomach open. "We went home and called the vet to tell him what we had found. Then we prayed all night."

Rose shares her very moving personal prayer to God that evening. "I've always felt in my heart that the Lord was part of me," she attests, "and I've always talked directly to Him. So I said, 'God, please take the pain away from her and bring it to me. I will take on Princess's suffering.' I also told Him that if He did decide to take Princess, to open his arms, hold her tight, then let her run free in heaven."

The following morning, a jangling telephone jarred the family awake. Rose still recalls how reluctant she was to answer it. She was expecting it to be bad news about Princess. But instead, she was in for a pleasant surprise.

"It was the vet, and he said that, incredibly, Princess had made it through the night and was doing very well.

The bleeding had stopped and he did not believe surgery was required."

An exuberantly joyful Rose knew that her prayers had been answered. "How else could a dog with its stomach torn apart make such a swift recovery? She was bleeding badly. She was in shock. You could have cut off her leg and she wouldn't have known it. She was literally at death's door. My husband and I didn't think surgery could save her."

Rose's first words to the veterinarian were, "Thank God. When can I come get her?"

"Right now, if you'd like," the veterinarian replied.

When she and Jay arrived at the animal clinic, Princess was well but too weak to walk. "We carried her to the car, took her home, and fed her by hand. In a couple of weeks, she was back to her old self. She had been saved."

Princess lived for six more happy and healthy years. "She died peacefully in our arms. But I'm not unhappy. God had saved her life until He wanted to take her.

"To this day, I can still feel her around the house—especially in the place she would lie down to sleep. I believe she is running free in heaven and is our little creature angel."

Rose has words of advice for anyone experiencing the agony of having a seriously ill or injured pet: "Believe in God. Open your heart and pray to Him," she declares. "He will do the right thing when you ask Him.

"And if He does take your pet home to heaven, just know that your beautiful animal will be happy there. I really believe it. I know that's where Princess is right now."

5 . A Guide Dog Gets a
New Leash on Life

WHEN Park, a seven-and-a-half-year-old Seeing Eye dog, was scheduled for abdominal surgery, his partially blind owner, Len Boulter, turned to the Scriptures of his faith.

The seventy-one-year-old Salt Lake City, Utah, resident and former marine states that there are "numerous incidents in our church history where animals have been given special blessings." So the evening before the Labrador retriever's scheduled surgery, he and his wife prayed fervently for one.

Len proclaims that what transpired the following day was proof not only that miracles can happen, but that God does not have a blind spot when it comes to granting mercy to His four-legged creatures.

• • •

There's a regular morning ritual which Len Boulter and Edith, his wife of more than fifty years, always enjoy performing, one which reinforces what Len already knows about his guide dog, Park—that he is an especially sensitive and intelligent animal.

Just before breakfast, the Boulters take time to kneel down on the kitchen floor and say their morning prayers. They do this knowing full well that the eighty-five-pound cinnamon-colored Lab is lurking about impatiently waiting to be fed.

"This is a dog that's never without a hearty appetite—especially in the morning," Len says laughingly. "Of course, Park knows that we keep his food in the kitchen; he's always in there bugging me to get his food out for him.

"But he also knows he's not allowed to come into the kitchen during our prayer time, so he'll stand at the threshold and watch us. And when I tell him, 'We have to say our prayers first,' I believe that he understands every word I say. He'll go away and get on his bed and wait until we finish praying. As soon as we're done, he's back with his nose in the kitchen."

Smart? You bet, says Len, who was not born blind but suffers from a degenerative eye disease. He often wonders how he ever got along without this clever guide dog, who on several occasions has kept him from serious harm.

Len recalls the time before 1995 when he was without a guide dog. Back then, the tall Len thought that it would be too costly for him to own such a dog. He also believed he wouldn't qualify for a Seeing Eye dog because he wasn't completely sight-impaired.

He changed his mind after reading an article about a partially blind woman who owned such a guide dog. Len contacted the not-for-profit Guide Dogs for the Blind in San Rafael, California, where he learned that he was, indeed, eligible for a canine companion. The organization has been providing guide dogs to financially strapped sight-impaired people free or at a low cost since 1942.

"Not only did I qualify for a guide dog," he declares, "but they even paid for my transportation to their guide dog training school in California so that I could learn how to handle one of these animals. They paid for my housing, the whole bit.

"Before I left home, I prayed very fervently that they would match me with the right dog," he recalls. Prayers, he notes, have always played an important role in his life—from the time he was a youngster growing up in Salt Lake City to the present day.

Upon arriving at the Guide Dogs for the Blind school, Len was given a week of training on the care and handling of these special canines. After he completed the course, the day came when he was to be introduced to his future guide dog.

"I remember that the trainer brought Park to my room, and from the first time I met him, we just bonded immediately," he says. "It was a match made in heaven, and I truly believe that God created this guide dog just for me."

He can still recall how the two-year-old Lab gazed intently at him. "It was like he had recognized me— like we had known each other all our lives. He came over to me, looked me over, sniffed me, and from then on we were buddies."

Len's first impression of Park was that "this is a very friendly and very calm dog. He was well behaved from the beginning. Even today, people are amazed at how well behaved he is in restaurants or wherever we go.

He just never makes any kind of commotion."

Len goes on to further extol Park's virtues. "He likes people very much. If he does have any fault, it's that he sometimes gets distracted because he likes people—and other animals—so much. But he's very obedient for the most part and very dependable."

Today, Len has become the Utah representative for Guide Dogs for the Blind. He often speaks before groups of visually impaired people, always encouraging sight-impaired members of his audience to obtain a guide dog. " 'How much is your life worth?' I always ask the people I speak to. Then I tell the story of how Park once literally saved my own life from an oncoming car I didn't see."

Len and Park are inseparable now, and they've formed a very strong bond. So understandably, Len was very upset when Park suddenly became ill in February 2000. "He started to throw up," Len explains. "It wasn't a continual thing—just periodically. Sometimes, during the night, we would hear him."

One particular afternoon when Len was attending a meeting at the Guide Dogs for the Blind's Oregon campus, Park's condition seemed to worsen.

"I took him into the clinic that's on the campus, and the vet checked him over. He couldn't seem to find anything wrong, so I took Park home and he continued to throw up. He still wasn't all right.

"A month later, while I was at another Guide Dogs for the Blind meeting, this time at the San Rafael campus, he was throwing up a lot again. I immediately took him to their clinic."

Park was examined by veterinarian Autumn Davidson, who did a thorough workup on the dog, including

X rays. The X rays showed that a foreign object was lodged in Park's stomach.

"Dr. Davidson wasn't sure if it was a rock or a bottle cap," Len recalls, "but she said it had obviously been there for about two months. She said, 'I think we better do surgery.' "

Len was devastated by the news. "I had brought Park to the clinic on a Friday afternoon, and Dr. Davidson scheduled Park for surgery the following Monday morning. On Saturday, I was supposed to bring him in for more X rays."

That night, Len called Edith to inform her about the situation. His wife said she would join him as quickly as possible. Len hung up the phone and got right down on his knees in his hotel room and began to pray for Park.

Meanwhile, at home, Edith was doing the same before leaving to join her husband. "We both prayed very fervently for most of the night that he would be all right," he attests.

The following morning, Len brought Park back to the animal medical clinic for further X rays. That's when he believes a miracle occurred. "They took more X rays and there was nothing there!" Len exclaims.

"Dr. Davidson walked into the clinic and said, 'Len, I don't know how to tell you this, but whatever was there is gone.' Then she showed me the X ray. Everything was clean.

"The doctor couldn't believe it, and needless to say, I was overjoyed.

"It couldn't have been anything else but an act of God. I don't think there's any question about it."

Not wanting to take any chances, Len stayed over

the weekend and brought Park back to the clinic on Monday morning for some final precautionary tests.

"Park was given more X rays, but the results were the same," he declares. "Nothing could be found in his stomach or his bowels. The vet said to me, 'Take him home. He's fine.' "

Nowadays, whenever the subject of Park's remarkable recovery comes up, Len has this to say about it: "I think it shows that dogs definitely have their place in heaven. The teachings of our church are correct when they suggest that God's mercy is not reserved for human beings alone.

"Animals are a creation of God and they respond to prayer. There are numerous incidents in our church history where animals have been given special blessings."

For anyone whose pet is scheduled for surgery, Len advises that prayers be said for that animal. "Make sure it's getting the best medical attention, and then pray on its behalf. Prayer is essential. It's the key that can save your pet's life."

6 . The Haunted Racehorse

CARLA Person, a Shamanic healer and animal communicator, has for more than fourteen years been working with her Native American spirit guides to help heal animals and humans alike.

The Venta, Oregon, resident, who teaches marketing at the University of Oregon, recalls that of all the cases she has been involved with over the years, the one which stands out in her mind involves a racehorse with a bizarre personality disorder.

Skip to Fame, a retired fifteen-year-old Thoroughbred known to horse-racing fans all along the East Coast, could at one moment be sweet and gentle and, at the next, suddenly turn violent.

When, in desperation, the horse's owner turned to Carla for assistance, the shamanic healer and her spirit guides discovered the startling reason behind the Thoroughbred's unusual behavior.

Today, the handsome chestnut bay gelding with the small white star on its forehead is a much calmer animal. He is enjoying his pastures of plenty thanks to Carla's ministrations and the help of otherworldly spirit guides.

. . .

Carla Person seems to operate comfortably in two entirely separate realities. By day, she teaches e-commerce and Web marketing at the University of Oregon. When she is not teaching, Carla is kept busy practicing her psychic skills as an animal communicator and shamanic healer.

A graduate of the Foundation for Shamanic Studies, the forty-three-year-old former marketing executive says her attraction to "core shamanism"—which utilizes spiritual healing practices from a variety of native cultures around the world—was the result of a long search for a spiritual practice that she could relate to.

"I was raised in a family that understood Christianity but never went to church," she declares. "Over the years, I tried a lot of different religions, and even studied religion and philosophy. I got a strong Western education in religion, but I still couldn't quite figure out where I fit in. Then my sister recommended that I see a woman who practiced shamanism—this was in 1984 or 1985—so I did. That visit completely changed my life."

From that moment on, she began a serious study of shamanism. It was about four years ago that she decided to apply what she had learned to helping animals as well as people.

"I've always very much been an animal person," she emphasizes, "and I discovered that there are really very

few shamans who work with animals. I thought that
with my special skills I could help."

Since then, Carla says that she and her spirit guides
have participated in the healing of many different animals—from goats to dogs to horses. "Like people, animals have helping spirits," she explains. "And the
spirits I work with often provide healing power and
comfort to my animal clients."

One of Carla's most intriguing cases involved a retired racehorse with a schizophrenic personality. Skip
to Fame first came to her attention about a year and a
half ago, when Carla received a letter from the chestnut
bay's upstate New York owner, Mary Arena.

The horse owner wrote Carla that Skip to Fame had
a Doctor Jekyll and Mister Hyde temperament. She
added that if the gelding could not be cured of his
aggressiveness, he might have to be put down. "I want
you to do a healing for Skip to Fame," Arena continued. "He's been with me for seven years. I actually
bought him for my daughter, who is an aspiring horse
trainer, but I felt a strong connection with him from
the start, and felt that he was meant to be with me. He
appears to be a normal, high-strung Thoroughbred, but
he started to unravel emotionally shortly before coming
here."

The letter went on:

"There's a Pandora's box of fears that he seems to
be holding inside of himself. He's become more and
more out of control and extremely dangerous. He's a
horse of extremes. A warm, friendly, charismatic animal who, at times, becomes untouchable and will attack any person or animal he can get to."

Skip to Fame's owner explained the various attempts

she had made to resolve her horse's problems, including several sessions with an animal communicator—someone who psychically "talks" with nonhuman creatures.

She told Carla that all of those efforts had proved futile. "Nothing that's been done could break through Skip's wall of aggression that he built. He wanted nothing to do with humans."

Carla, who owns several horses herself and declares that "horses are everything to me in my life," says she felt compelled to help. She then turned to her Native American spirit guides for assistance.

"When people ask me to do shamanic healing work for their animals, there are two basic things I do," she explains. "First, I enter a state of nonordinary reality. I 'journey' to the animal and 'speak' with it.

"There I get impressions of the animal's past and let the owner know what the animal's memories and current impressions are. In that journey, I also enter the animal's body and see if there is any pain or injury.

"Secondly, I ask my helping spirits—they specialize in animals, including horses—if the animal needs further help. I also ask these spirits to heal the hurt animal and learn if there is any specific treatment that would be good for me to pursue."

. . .

It was a beautiful summer day when Carla embarked upon her shamanic journey to heal Skip to Fame. She began, as she always does, with meditation and prayer. "I pray a lot before I get started," she emphasizes. "I pray to all the spirits that I work with, and I pray to the spirits that they work with. And as you work your way up the chain, you get to the Great Spirit—God."

Having attained her desired altered state, Carla encountered the spirit guide who has often worked with her in the past. "I can't tell you exactly who this guide is," she states, "except to say that he is a Native American who lived about a hundred and fifty years ago. I know that he was once a great horseman. After I explained the situation to him, he led me to other guides who are specifically responsible for the healing of horses. I remember that my spirit guide then set up a healing circle. It's in that sacred circle that the healing work begins."

Carla says she watched with fascination as her spirit guide then "called in a huge band of angels and a bunch of other spirits who I had never met before. These were spirits that he had worked with in the past—all of his teachers and their friends. We had some pretty serious help there." She chuckles.

When the guides were ready, Skip to Fame's spirit was invited to enter the sacred circle. Then Carla's guide began to "converse" with the horse's spirit. What he discovered was a bit of a surprise to her.

"My guide found that he was talking to *two* people! He was talking to the horse and he was talking to this raging, violent, and insane stable hand who had inhabited the horse's body.

"This was a stable hand who had been murdered over a drug deal or something. He was running with a bad crowd and got himself into a lot of trouble.

"This soul didn't quite believe he was dead, and wanted to keep running with the bad guys. So he lodged himself inside this sweet racehorse, who would

be calm and gentle one moment, and in the next, viciously attack people."

Although Carla acknowledges that to anyone not familiar with the world of psychic phenomena, all of this
may seem a bit far-fetched. But to her, it makes perfect
sense because this is the world in which shamans have
operated since time immemorial.

Carla also learned from her spirit guides that Skip
to Fame's possessing spirit had, while alive, abused the
horse. This, she contends, was one reason why the
horse would sometimes shy away from people.

Once the ostensible cause of the gelding's problems
was revealed, Carla says the next step was to coax the
inhabiting spirit out of the retired Thoroughbred. "Shamans can perform the critical function of helping souls
who have died," she explains. "Sometimes when an
animal or person dies suddenly, unexpectedly, the soul
doesn't know it's dead, and it hangs out here rather
than moving on to the light. This can be a problem for
the soul and for us here in ordinary reality."

Carla says that while in that astral space, she and
her guides tried to make the stablehand's spirit understand that he was dead. "We helped him to move on
to the light, where he would find peace and healing.
We were finally able to return the spirit to that part of
the afterworld where it belonged."

When Carla called Skip to Fame's owner and reported her experience, she says that the gelding's
owner was not very surprised. "She knew that Skip had
been abused—he showed the physical signs of that,"
Carla says. "And she was also aware that in cases of
possession, there are severe personality changes. It all
seemed to make sense to her."

Was Carla herself surprised by what she learned during her journey? She shrugs and smiles at the question. "I'm rarely surprised by anything that happens in this state," she attests. "Every case is different. When I'm in this state of nonordinary reality, everything seems weird."

Some weeks later, Carla received another letter from Skip to Fame's owner, one which she says brought her great pleasure. She reads from the letter:

Dear Carla:
     This has been a most fascinating experience for me and Skip. There are subtle and definite changes in him. He is a horse now with a different energy about him.
     The wariness in his disposition and the intensity are gone. He is feeling a new level of confidence. I think it will take some time for us both to get used to the *new* Skip. . . . He's normal now. . . .

"It was a happy solution to a horse's sadness!" Carla exclaims. "Sometimes the changes are dramatic as a result of a Shamanic journey and sometimes they're small. I'd say that this one was pretty dramatic . . ."

7 . A Pastor's Prayers Are Answered

FOR Sonya, a part Siberian husky/Samoyed, satisfying her sweet tooth nearly cost her her life.

When Sonya snuck into a bedroom and devoured a package of chocolate-covered Reese's Peanut Butter Cups that she found there, the dog suffered a severe physical reaction which sent her into convulsions and left her barely able to walk.

At one point, Sonya was so ill that her veterinarian recommended she be put to sleep.

Fortunately for Sonya, however, she had a Baptist minister for an owner who knew exactly what needed to be done to save the dog's life. The Reverend Lannie Dowell, pastor of a small church in Maryland, turned to prayer to save her critically ill pet.

Reverend Dowell is firmly convinced that Sonya went on to live an active and healthy life until she was sixteen years old because of her spiritual treatment. "God's Spirit took over the healing," she declares, "and opened the way for Sonya to make a full recovery."

■ ■ ■

There's a small church located in Columbia, Maryland, known as the Zion's Gate Baptist Church. What is very special about this church is its dynamic sixty-year-old pastor, the Reverend Lannie Dowell.

For the past sixteen years, Reverend Dowell has extended her healing ministry not only to people who are ill but to animals as well. Her animal ministry was inspired by the spiritual healing of her own dog, and years later, by the grief she experienced over its death.

"Sonya was a vibrant gift to our household," Reverend Dowell declares, "and I wanted to sustain and comfort others whose animals may be lost, injured, or in pain. I know that my faith in God sustained Sonya when she was ill, and that He can help heal other animals as well."

Today, in addition to her busy church schedule, Reverend Dowell operates an on-line chaplaincy in which she offers prayer and counseling via the Internet to anyone who has an ailing pet or is mourning the loss of one.

The Baptist minister does not consider this an unusual ministry. "There are quite a few ministers who will tell you that as children, they had experiences of burying dead birds, or dead squirrels, or dead cats before they even knew there was a call of God on their lives," she explains.

"They were conducting their childlike versions of funerals, and I think this was their preparation for having sympathy and respect for animals when they grew up and entered the church."

Reverend Dowell began her own preaching ministry

in 1983. Her mission in life, she says, has always been "healing and deliverance. God has a special ministry for each individual," she continues, "and the purpose for our lives is placed in us when we're still in our mother's womb.

"But I can only heal or deliver a person or an animal from harm if God wants it so. He has given us all healing gifts, but we can't change an event until He says so."

Recalling her childhood, the pastor says she has always had an interest in helping animals who were in trouble. "My family took in just about every stray," she laughingly shares.

"We had all kinds of dogs running around the house all the way through my teenage years. Even when they proliferated, we wouldn't get rid of any of them. I always had this affinity for animals—and people."

Her story of Sonya's miraculous recovery begins in the late 1970s "when my husband went to the local animal shelter to get a blue-eyed malamute that was being featured in the newspaper.

"Well, you can imagine my surprise when instead, he returned with a six-month-old part–Siberian husky/ Samoyed puppy in tow, named Sonya. So Sonya made her entrance into our lives.

"She made her acquaintance with our children, who were very young at the time. And she made her way into our home and hearts. We all settled into a brand-new, welcome friendship."

Reverend Dowell says it was in 1984 that Sonya became suddenly ill. By now, Sonya was a mature dog and the mother of her own litter. The illness was a mystery because no one knew that the dog had come across a bag of chocolate covered Reese's Peanut Butter Cups and devoured them all.

That need to satisfy a sweet tooth set off a near-fatal allergic reaction. "Only later did we find out how deadly chocolate is to some animals—that it could kill them," she explains. "We didn't know what had happened to Sonya at the time. All I know is that the results of that chocolate binge are something terrible to behold.

"We noticed that her hair was starting to fall out, her skin became scaly, she smelled like tar, and her legs would lock up in such a way that she was unable to walk. She lost a lot of weight and would go into convulsions."

A trip to the animal hospital resulted in a lot of tests but no cure for what ailed the dog. "Because we didn't know about the chocolate at the time, we didn't say anything to the veterinarian. The vet ended up treating her for malnutrition and said she would probably have to be put to sleep."

Not only the veterinarian but several fellow ministers and friends who came to Reverend Dowell's house to help her pray for the sick dog recommended that Sonya be destroyed. "They would come over and see Sonya in such bad shape—she would suddenly squeal as her back legs locked up—that they couldn't stand to see the animal suffering," she says. "So they told me to put her out of her misery."

However, as a dedicated Christian and animal lover who grew up in Baltimore surrounded by a household full of pets, Reverend Dowell says there was no way she would have a dog or anyone else killed.

What Reverend Dowell did instead was turn to

prayer. "You start with God when an animal is ill," she declares. "And while you continue to do everything you can to help that animal—including medical care—you continue to pray and walk with God and talk with Him through the entire ordeal. Everything begins and ends with prayer."

Reverend Dowell remembers beginning her healing work on Sonya with a firm conviction in her heart that if God wanted this dog to live, He would manage to effect a healing.

"I handled her, stroked her, talked to her, and prayed for her," she says. "The people who came over to pray for Sonya did the same. There wasn't any outward 'showing' the way some healers do," she explains. "I quietly let the Spirit lead. I realized it wasn't I who was healing Sonya, but God's Spirit. It was God who had His hand on my hand. I was just an available and willing vessel."

Whenever Sonya showed signs of distress, Reverend Dowell says she would place hands on her. "I would hear her squeal and I would get up and walk over to her and lay hands on her. I would quietly pray. I had belief and faith that God would heal her."

Remarkably, the dog who seemed to be at death's doorstep, gradually began to respond to her owner's spiritual ministrations. "Each time I laid hands on Sonya and prayed for her, she would get up and feel better," the pastor smilingly asserts.

"I mean this dog's legs would lock, she would go into convulsions, and then start shaking. I would lay hands on her and pray, and within minutes she was up and running around. It was a miracle, and only God could have done it," she declares with conviction in her voice.

But there was more to come. "The first miracle was that she didn't immediately die from eating all that chocolate," Reverend Dowell continues. "The second was that we brought Sonya to another vet who eventually discovered what was basically wrong with the dog—most especially that she lacked the proper amount of zinc.

"He prescribed a medication and Sonya began to thrive. She lived until her final demise some years later, looking the very picture of health even on the very day and hour she breathed her last!

"If I had given up and had Sonya euthanized as the first veterinarian and some of my friends had suggested, she wouldn't have been with us for years after. But God sustained her. I also know that if I hadn't put hands on her, she may have lingered, but she would have suffered terribly. It all was a sequence of miracles."

Sonya went on to live until age sixteen, passing away in February 1998. Although she grieved at her loss, the minister also recalls thanking God "for delivering her from this body of death to life, and allowing me to be present at the crossing-over."

It was Sonya's death that prompted Reverend Dowell to reach out more actively to other pet owners who might have recently lost a beloved pet. "I learned another important life lesson at that time—how much people can suffer at the loss of one of their animal friends. It was through my own suffering that it occurred to me that I could become a chaplain for other pet owners.

"I began to understand that people can suffer as much from the loss of a pet as they can from losing one of their relatives. The agony and the pain is the same. Pet owners feel a responsibility to support and help their pets, and when an animal dies, they feel somehow guilty for that death."

During her counseling sessions, Reverend Dowell says, she emphasizes that there is nothing wrong with expressing grief over the loss of a beloved pet. "Through the grief comes the release," she declares. "You have to have that expression of grief and recognize it as such."

She also advises bereaved pet owners to take their time with the grieving process. "It's okay to mourn for an animal for one or two years—or even longer. Even after so much time you may only be at the beginning of relieving yourself of the grief or any guilt you may be feeling."

One thing which she continually emphasizes is that "God does love all animals, and these departed animal souls will find a home in heaven. We have the illustrations of God's love for animals all through the Bible," she says, "starting with the story of Noah and the ark."

The minister adds that whenever she is asked the difficult question of why God has allowed a pet to die, her answer is that "everything that is born will die. That's a reality of life. Death comes to us all.

"I don't get too deep into this discussion, which can lead into the whole theology of life after death. My purpose is to try to give the person who contacts me immediate relief and release in the moment. I try to give the grieving pet owner encouragement and hope so that they will be able to get on with their lives."

On the question of whether animals have souls, Reverend Dowell asserts with no hesitation that they most certainly do. "Every living thing—everything that breathes—has a soul," she attests. "God placed the breath of life in animals, in human beings—even in plants."

Since Sonya's passing, Reverend Dowell says she learned to console herself with her loss by focusing on the many happy times she spent with her pet over the years. Sonya, she emphasizes, has now experienced the ultimate healing, because her soul has returned to God.

"That's something for anyone with a pet friend who is dying to remember—although they don't want to hear it," she says. "We want our loved ones—whether it's a pet or a close relative—to be here. But you need to know that going to God is the only place where we can really be healed or at peace."

Summing it all up, Reverend Dowell says: "When Sonya was ill after eating all those chocolates, God showed me His healing powers. By witnessing that, I experienced a blessing as well.

"God has always wanted me to preach and pastor, and this helped strengthen my personal relationship with the Lord so that I would never doubt Him."

8 . The Cat with Eleven Lives

IT'S pretty much assumed that most cats have nine lives, but Mary Arthur, a freelance writer, part-time astrology teacher, and animal intuitive counselor, believes that her late cat, Spooky, had a few extra ones.

"Twice that I know of this cat survived when the odds were down to nothing," the Roseburg, Oregon, resident asserts. "She always amazed me."

The first time that Spooky narrowly avoided death was when a friendly cat fed her and kept the feral feline from starving. Some years later, when she was diagnosed with a fatal form of feline leukemia and given only a week to live, Spooky again beat the odds.

"This is a cat who I'm sure had eleven lives," Mary declares with conviction. "Spooky was a cat who was blessed by God."

. . .

Mary Arthur's life is filled with animals. A visitor to her small farmhouse in rural Oregon, where she raises wool for spinning, can find a menagerie of cats, dogs, rabbits, chickens, goats, sheep—and even a baby lamb that was abandoned by its mother.

That's because the fifty-year-old freelance writer and part-time astrologer says she's making up for a childhood in Fairbanks, Alaska, where there was practically not a single variety of animal to be found.

"I always felt really animal deprived," she says, laughing. "There just wasn't a lot of animals besides the usual pets when I was growing up there. I think I had just two cats and one dog all those years."

Today, Mary's farm seems to be a magnet for wayward animals. "Stray animals find us, lost cats find us," she says. No matter what kind of lost or abandoned four-footed creature shows up at her doorstep, Mary and her husband, Ray, are unable to turn it away.

In addition to being a soft touch for wayward animals, Mary has an intuitive sense about them—a psychic gift she has been aware of since childhood. When her neighbors' pets are not feeling well, it's Mary whom they call upon for a little advice.

"I also teach astrology and beginning intuition, and at times I've taught people how to work with their animals—how to take care of them, the proper foods, that kind of thing," she says. "It's mostly based on my intuitive abilities, and it's kind of become a profession for me.

"Some people kid me that this close feeling I have with animals is 'misplaced maternal instinct,' " she continues, laughing at the notion, "but I've always felt in touch with the feelings of animals. I just love animals. They're more honest in their relationships with people, and I enjoy their company. You don't have to put on airs for them."

Mary displays a wonderful sense of humor as she spins story after story about her family of sheep, goats, rabbits, "and a few silly chickens."

Her favorite story, however, is about Spooky, who for many years lived a charmed life. The account, however, begins with another of Mary's many cats— Squeak—who first led her to discover the feral feline.

"It was 1986 and Ray and I began to notice that Squeak, whose mother was killed on the highway, was bringing mice it had captured to a crawl hole under our house," Mary relates. "One day, this absolutely skin-and-bones adult cat—there was nothing there—came out from under the house.

"We figured out that Squeak was feeding this starving cat. Every day Squeak would bring a mouse to her. We live about a half a block from the highway, and people are always releasing animals from their cars. I think this cat was a pet that someone wanted to get rid of."

The cat that cautiously emerged from the crawl hole beneath Mary's house was white with black spots and quite wild. "You couldn't get close to her," she says. "You'd catch a glimpse of her and then she'd be gone."

When Mary first saw the cat, whom she eventually named Spooky, she thought it was remarkable that the wild feline had survived at all. "She looked like a cat that had been in a concentration camp. She looked half-dead. So we started putting cat food out under the house because we didn't want her to starve to death."

It took four months of continual and patient coaxing by Mary's husband to convince Spooky to emerge per-

manently from her hiding place and take up family life.
"Ray finally got her to come over to him, and she allowed us to bring her into the house—but she still
looked ratty."

Almost from the very beginning, Spooky began to
cotton up to Mary. For the first time in months, the cat
began purring with contentment. "She would snuggle
up to me and I could still feel all of her bones, she was
so thin. Her black hair was smooth, but her white hair
looked like a porcupine. She looked really terrible."

It was the start of a long and happy relationship between Spooky and her new owners. Then another of
her nine lives was put to the test when Spooky fell
suddenly ill.

"This was in the early 1990s," Mary recalls. "She
started losing weight, and had dropped her weight to
almost what it was when we first found her. We didn't
know what was wrong. So I took her to the Baily Veterinary Clinic. The vet diagnosed her with feline leukemia, and also a form of cat AIDS."

The diagnosis shocked her. "I just couldn't believe
it," she asserts. "Then the vet said he wanted to put
her down because she looked so bad." Mary, however,
balked at that idea.

There was no way she was going to have Spooky
put to sleep without first trying other ways to save her
life. "I told the vet that I would take Spooky home and
see what I could do to make her feel better."

Mary can still recall the skeptical look on the veterinarian's face, and how much that look angered her.
"I said, 'If this was your cat, you wouldn't want to put
her down without trying.' And he didn't have a word
to say."

When Mary returned home with her ailing cat, she immediately began a regimen that included "plenty of love and affection" along with a heavy dose of prayer.

"I started to give her nice warm baths in the sink to stimulate her blood circulation and keep her skin nice and supple, and I added cod-liver oil to her diet. I petted her a lot and gave her a lot of reassurance."

Mary, who grew up in a religious household where prayer was part of everyday life, recollects that "each night I would hold Spooky against my heart like you do a baby. I would pray to God to save this beautiful animal. I gave all the encouragement I could to Spooky, and then I turned her over to a Higher Power. I said, 'God, this is my kitty. Don't take her from me.'"

Within a week, Mary began to notice improvement in Spooky's condition. "She went from being on the verge of death to recovering absolutely beautifully," Mary declares. "This cat who the vet wanted to put down lived another eight years—well into old age. She died at home very peacefully."

Spooky's recovery was nothing less than a miracle to Mary. "She wasn't expected to survive at all," she emphasizes, "and yet she survived with absolutely no symptoms of either the leukemia or the AIDS. It was amazing to me that twice since we got her, Spooky had gone from practically nothing to being alive and healthy."

The powerful effect of prayer does not surprise Mary at all. "I totally believe in it," she affirms. "You never know what's going to happen. I believe that God responded to it and kept Spooky around for a reason that I'm not aware of. She was around for a long time, and

I'm very much appreciative that she didn't die when
she was expected to."

As a result of her own experience, Mary urges anyone with a seriously ill cat never to give up hope. "Always think positively and believe in the best," she
attests. "Give the animal permission to do what it
wants to do—whether it wants to stay or go on—and
pray. Pray from your heart. That's the main thing."

9 . Wings and a Prayer

SIVAJI Narayanasamy, head chef at New York City's Sanctuary Restaurant, does more than prepare sumptuous dishes at the popular East Village vegetarian eatery. The Malaysian-born chef is also a Reiki energy healer, massage therapist, and an active member of the Interfaith League of Devotees, a not-for-profit religious group that practices Krishna consciousness, a Hindu-based religion.

When a friend suddenly had to return home to Europe, he left behind a parakeet named Leo for Sivaji to care for. Sivaji and the bird grew to be such trusting friends that the chef often would not lock Leo's cage and allow the parakeet to fly freely around his apartment.

There was a night when Sivaji returned home to find Leo looking listless and, apparently, quite ill. When the one-year-old bird failed to respond to medical treatment, Sivaji says he turned to his spiritual tradition for a cure.

What transpired in the hours that followed did not really surprise Sivaji, who emphasizes that Hinduism has taught for thousands of years that animals as well as people have souls, and that even birds can respond positively to the chanting of God's holy name.

. . .

Having grown up in a suburb called Ipoh, located just outside of Malaysia's capital city, Kuala Lumpur, Sivaji recalls that he and his family always had dogs and other pets running around the house

"I've always loved animals," says the handsome chef with the serene smile. "I remember that there were always birds flying around outside our house. I think that's how I ended up with Leo—a friend of mine from Austria had to return home on banking business, and he knew I was a big bird lover."

Sivaji laughingly relates that the friend "packed up everything for his trip except for the parakeet. I went over there the night before he and his wife left, and he said he didn't know what to do with the parakeet, because nobody wanted him. So I agreed to take him back with me."

Since Sivaji had never owned a bird before, getting familiar with his new pet was, at first, a bit of a challenge. "The first two or three weeks Leo was kind of scared of me, because I was this dark-skinned foreigner," he quips. "But then he started to like me. I would just give him his freedom in my room for two or three hours, and let him fly around. Sometimes I'd let him fly around all day. He would go back to his cage whenever he was hungry, and he would patiently wait for me to feed him."

In the course of a year, Leo became so trusting and attached to Sivaji "that as soon as I called his name he'd come to me. He would land on my shoulder and play with me. He was a very friendly and social bird."

One night Sivaji returned to his apartment and immediately sensed that something was wrong with his pet bird. "I wasn't exactly sure what was happening to him," he explains, "but he was so weak that he was falling asleep all the time. I knew that when birds get sick, they sleep all day like someone with a fever. He was sitting in one corner of his cage and would never move. He was losing feathers and wouldn't eat."

Sivaji rushed over to a nearby pet shop, where he was given some herbal preparations to help perk the bird up. "I tried all the supplements and they didn't work—he was still the same."

Late one night Sivaji decided to try a different approach before taking the bird to the veterinarian. "I reached into the cage and took Leo into my hands," he relates. "The bird seemed to be very scared and didn't want to be touched. And then I started chanting Hare Krishna for about a half hour."

Sivaji explains that Krishna is how God's name is pronounced in the ancient Sanskrit language of India, and that Hindus believe that chanting is the best means for evoking God's favors. "We also believe that animals are our brothers and sisters—not only in this lifetime, but in many lifetimes—and have souls just like human beings do. So I prayed for Leo.

"I wasn't praying to God to keep the bird alive," he says. "I was just asking that if the bird had to die, to let it die peacefully and not to suffer. I remember praying for Leo like I would for a human being, because this bird was a good friend of mine."

Sivaji gently held Leo in his hand as he chanted God's name. The repetitive sound of the words seemed to lull the bird into a state of deep relaxation.

"There wasn't any instant miracle or anything like that," Sivaji says. "I finally got sleepy myself and put Leo back into his cage. When I woke up the next morning, I was really surprised—Leo was looking very good!

"I took the cover off the cage, opened it, and Leo went shooting out and started flying around." He laughs at that memory. "He was back to normal. I felt sure that he had recovered because of my prayers."

Sivaji, who practices the Japanese form of energy healing known as Reiki, says he has read many articles about how prayer can help people who are physically, psychologically, or spiritually ill. He is now convinced it works for animals as well. "I don't know if Leo was suffering from a physical or emotional problem, I just knew the next morning he was suddenly better."

For other pet owners with a sick animal on their hands, Sivaji advises them to pray. "It doesn't matter if you know how to pray or not—it's just the thought that counts," he asserts. "Just ask God to help and He will, because He's present in everyone's heart. Just sincerely ask for His help."

After that miraculous healing, Sivaji says Leo went on to live an active bird's life for eight more months, dying peacefully one evening of natural causes. "I really miss him because he was very attached to me, and I felt the same about him," he declares. "I always treated him as I would a human being."

To illustrate the close level of attachment between the two of them, Sivaji relates the story of Leo's passing in a voice tinged with sadness. "It was Christmas Day and that morning for about two hours I was playing with Leo," he recollects. "He was flying around and playing with me and having fun.

"I came back home later that night, and the first thing I wanted to check on was Leo. I looked into his cage and Leo stared at me for a few seconds in a strange way. I said, 'Whoa! Why is this bird staring at me this way?' Then Leo went over to where his water was, drank two sips, and then just fell down dead."

Sivaji says he held the bird in his hand and chanted, but this time Leo could not escape death's grip. "He died in a very peaceful manner. But what I find most remarkable is that he waited a whole day until he could say good-bye to me before he died. That's still so sad for me to think about."

10 . God's Little Miracle Dog

CRUELLY tied by its neck to a tree with a wire hanger, wounded by rifle pellets, and tortured, the little black chow's odds of survival did not seem high when Shari Ferguson and her father came upon him while walking their dogs in the Clearlake, Texas, woods.

Worsening matters, Bear, as the dog was later called, fled his rescuers despite his weakened condition, facing further trials while on the run.

But Shari, who operates a local animal-assisted therapy ministry, declares that Bear is a "miracle dog." How else could the chow have survived both these ordeals?

Her account of Bear's unusual rescue, and his subsequent battle to regain his health, is actually the story of a double miracle, one whose main character is a little black chow that was obviously touched by God.

• • •

Shari Ferguson has a special nickname for her canine buddy. "I call him God's Little Miracle all the time," she smilingly declares. "I gave him that nickname because of all he's been through.

"I just know it was a miracle that God kept him alive," she continues. "The way he was rescued and how he survived his various surgeries were all miracles. They were answers to my prayers and the prayers of others."

The thirty-nine-year-old computer programmer and founder of the Faithful Friends Animal-Assisted Therapy Ministry in Clearlake, Texas, located just south of Houston, recalls that it was a cold November day in 1994 when she and her father discovered the injured chow.

"My father and I decided to take a walk with our two dogs—a collie-shepherd and a husky," she relates. "It was something we did pretty regularly, and we liked to walk along the woods. This morning there was one area where we heard all this noise."

When Shari and her father investigated, they came across a disturbing sight. "There was this little black chow tied to a tree with a clothes hanger," she recalls, disgust registering in her voice. "He was wounded and apparently had been shot at. I think somebody was learning how to shoot, so they shot at him. We also think he was tortured while he was tied up."

Shari and her father tried to free the helpless dog, but not without some apprehension. "He was hurt and he was scared, and we weren't sure that he wouldn't bite us or our dogs while we were trying to get the wire off him."

In the midst of their efforts, however, something unexpected happened. "The hanger broke off from the
tree and the dog—despite all his wounds—ran off and
he wouldn't come close to us."

Concerned about the wounded runaway, Shari returned to the area each day for the next two weeks;
she brought food, treats, and water in an effort to entice
the chow closer. She hoped to capture Bear and bring
him home.

"I couldn't seem to get him," she relates. "When I
was walking with my other two dogs, he would come
close, but then he would move away. He just didn't
seem to trust people at all."

Shari had another concern about Bear. "The woods
were next to a highway, and I was afraid he'd get run
over," she says. "There's a lot of traffic on that road."

With Bear still on the loose, Shari decided one night
to call upon God for help. "I prayed all night to Him,
and I prayed whenever I was trying to get the dog,"
she asserts. "I would ask God to please not let him get
hurt."

While her prayers seemed to come naturally, Shari
admits there was a time when praying wasn't so easy
for her to do. Although she was raised Presbyterian,
churchgoing wasn't much of a family activity. "I didn't
even read the Bible until I was in college," she says.

The blond-haired, brown-eyed computer programmer says her spiritual life was renewed when she attended Texas A&M University to study finance. It was
there that she became involved with the Campus Cru-
sade for Christ. "I really started practicing Christianity," she asserts. "When I graduated and came back
home here, I got involved with the Baptist church."

With Bear still on the run, it was on God that Shari now fully depended for assistance. As the days passed, her prayers slowly began to be answered.

"Bear grew a little bit more trustful of me, but still not trustful enough to let me get too close," she recalls. "He would eat the food I gave him, but between bites he would look up to make sure I wasn't getting too near."

Then an event occurred which Shari believes was divinely inspired. "I was having some work done on my town house," she relates, "and we had the house open and the garage open for the construction workers to come through."

Shari says her collie-shepherd was tied up outside the garage to a ladder when a cat ran by. That's all the dog had to see. "Well, my dog started chasing after the cat and he was dragging the ladder behind him." She chuckles. "The collie-shepherd was running around the neighborhood causing quite a ruckus before returning back home.

"Apparently, the chow heard all this noise and became curious. He followed my collie-shepherd back home and walked right into my backyard." When Shari saw Bear entering her backyard, she could not believe her eyes. It was as if the runaway had been delivered by God right into her arms.

"That's how we were able to finally get him cornered," she says. "It was an answer to my prayers. I think this whole episode with my dog and the ladder was set up by God, and it was nothing short of a miracle how it ended with the chow following him right to us."

But Bear's problems weren't quite over. "It wasn't

easy to get the wire hanger off of his neck. It dug in so deeply into his throat that we couldn't cut it. We had to carefully untie it, and that took us a while because he still didn't trust us. He didn't know if we were pulling it tighter or what."

Despite the dog's anxiety, Shari remembers that Bear remained fairly calm, testifying to his gentle personality. Still, she feared the dog might have to be put to sleep. "I'd talked to some animal rescue people, and they told me that because of everything that he'd been through, he would never be able to be around humans again, so he needed to be put down."

But Shari says she hadn't gone through all this effort to rescue the chow just to have him killed. "We finally got the hanger off, and we took him to my vet," she relates. The prognosis wasn't a good one.

"It turned out that he had heartworms, parasites, gun pellet wounds, plus the problem with his throat. He also had some issues with his eyes, and the vet would have to operate on them."

When her veterinarian, Dr. Bobby Stevener, finished his examination of the chow, Shari was cautioned that the dog might not survive his injuries. "He said, 'I can't promise you that he's going to make it.' "

By now, it wasn't only Shari who was praying for Bear's recovery. "I think just about everyone who worked at the Pearland Veterinary Clinic was praying along with me," she declares. "They said he was such a cute little dog, so we were all praying that he would make it."

It took two years and a series of operations before Bear was completely out of danger. And not once during this long ordeal did Shari ever stop praying for the ailing chow.

Bear's complete recovery from all his injuries impressed everyone at the animal hospital, Shari recalls. "Dr. Stevener told me afterward that he was surprised how well Bear had come through.

"Later on, when he learned that Bear was assisting me with my ministry, he told me he was also surprised that Bear was doing so well around people, because he was so skittish and afraid of them."

But Bear always seemed to surprise everyone. For example, the first time she brought him home after his hospital stay, Shari was concerned that he wouldn't get along with her other two dogs. "I had two males already, so I wasn't sure they'd get along with a third male."

But the miracle dog who had survived abuse, gunshot wounds, and major surgery also managed to finesse his tense homecoming. "He wasn't feeling very well and he was so glad to have a place to stay," Shari recalls. "So he did the smartest thing he could have done—he just submitted to the other two dogs. I think he just walked in and rolled over," she laughingly relates.

It took another two years before Bear began to feel comfortable around people. "He didn't try to attack people, but he was afraid of them. He was extremely shy and would try to pull away from them."

What Shari hoped to do was eventually involve Bear in her animal-assisted therapy ministry, which she began in 1994 as an offshoot of her work with the local University Baptist Church.

"Over the years I was involved with several different

ministries—including a street ministry for kids," she explains, "but none of them was the type of ministry where you got to know the people very well. These people would come and go, and I'm more of a relationship type of person.

"What I really wanted to do was operate a program that involved both animals and the elderly. I was raised mostly by my grandmother. It was because of her that I really enjoyed being with senior adults."

Shari also grew up around animals, including puppies and an Australian shepherd. This love of animals and the elderly got her interested in animal-assisted therapy programs, where dogs and cats were brought into nursing homes, hospitals, and other institutions to help comfort patients.

"I told my pastor at the University Baptist Church that this was the kind of ministry I really wanted to start," she asserts, "and he told me to go for it, which I did."

Another reason why Shari wanted to start such a ministry was that it would allow her to spend more time with her two dogs, who were home alone a lot because of Shari's busy schedule. "I located some organizations that were doing animal-assisted therapy on a national level, and talked with them," she recalls. "They helped me to franchise their program locally."

Along with a partner, Shari launched the new ministry, which took off immediately. "We started growing from there. When we got big enough where we could do everything by ourselves, we began our own independent local group. We called it the Faithful Friends Animal-Assisted Therapy Ministry, and today, we have about a hundred and fifty volunteers out there visiting people in hospitals and other places."

When Shari felt that Bear could handle being around people, she decided to work up enough nerve to take him over to a local children's psychiatric hospital. The hospital worked with abused children, and over the years, Shari, as part of her Faithful Friends Animal-Assisted Therapy Ministry, would bring dogs there for the youngsters to play with.

When she arrived with Bear, the chow did not disappoint her. "In the first few minutes that I took him in there, one of the little boys came over to him, sat down next to him, and started petting him," Shari relates. "Bear started licking him and giving him doggy kisses. It was incredible. The child stayed with him the whole hour we were there on the visit.

"As we were leaving, one of the therapists came up to me and said, 'This is the first time we've seen that boy respond to anything or anybody.' Eventually, that little boy and that little dog became best of buds, and they teamed up whenever I visited the facility."

Shari says that therapists at the hospital utilized Bear as a tool to help this child to open up. "They'd have him explain what it would feel like to be the dog that was being abused and attacked," she relates. "He was able to talk about the dog's feelings but not his own. Through Bear he was able to finally release his own feelings."

Shari is firmly convinced that prayer was the key that made a happy ending for this story possible. "I know that God heard all those prayers because he kept Bear safe for the two weeks that he was running loose in traffic," she attests.

"I remember that my dad and I would always say, 'We can't believe he's running through all this traffic and he hasn't gotten hit by a car.' And the way he came into our backyard was nothing short of a miracle that was an answer to our prayers.

"It was also an answer to our prayers that he was saved through all his surgeries. And now, to see the way he works with these kids—that whole thing is nothing short of a miracle."

Shari believes that God's Little Miracle Dog is now being used by the Creator to "help create miracles in other people's lives—especially those of abused children. Now that he's recovered, he's touched so many people's lives," she declares.

"Bear's story will always be a reminder to me that it doesn't matter what you've been through, because God can make use of those experiences the way He's now using Bear to help others."

11 • A Miracle in the Foothills

BUTCH was an aptly named cat, barely two years old but tough as nails.

When the solid-gray-colored cat became lost for nearly a week in the foothills of the Colorado mountains, Beth White, organizer of a dalmatian rescue group in the Fort Collins area, feared the worst for her new pet. She was certain either the cold weather or coyotes would finish Butch off.

What Beth did not realize is that God had other plans for the feline runaway, and that his nine lives were far from used up. Just when things seemed most desperate, a most unusual occurrence took place, something which Beth describes as the "miracle in the foothills."

• • •

For more than thirty years, Beth White and her husband, Jack, a veterinarian who specializes in large-animal medicine, have lived on a four-hundred-acre ranch in the foothills of Colorado.

Over those years, Beth says she has observed many wonders and mysterious happenings in those remote foothills, but none that compares with the unusual events that took place in the winter of 1972 when Butch ran away from home.

Before getting into that story, Beth backtracks a bit to a time two years earlier, when she had recently arrived in Colorado from Anchorage, Alaska, where she was born and raised. She had come to Colorado to study veterinary medicine at Colorado State University.

Animals had always held a special place in her heart. "As a kid, I always loved them, and I grew up with a cat or two around the house. We also had Dachshunds. But I was especially horse-crazy. I read all the horse books I could get my hands on. I really wanted to be a veterinarian when I grew up."

Although Beth had her eyes set on entering Colorado State University's veterinary school, she quickly realized that she didn't have much of an aptitude for science, so she majored in history instead. "Instead of becoming a vet, I ended up marrying one," she quips. "So one way or another I've been surrounded by animals my whole life."

Even today, the fifty-year-old rancher and editorial assistant for the *Journal of Climate* sees that a special bond exists between her and the animal world. "Needy animals always seem to find me." She laughs. "God must say, 'Beth's not busy, let Me send her this animal or that animal that needs help.' It happens when I'm walking or even driving my car."

In 1989, that desire to assist helpless animals resulted in her organizing the Dalmatian Rescue of Colorado. She proudly notes that since its founding, the organization has rescued and placed well over 1,350 abandoned dals in foster homes.

Beth says her interest in dals began after meeting Jack, who used to breed them. "Nowadays," she adds, "I'm busier saving dalmatians than breeding them. I think of myself more as a rescuer than a breeder."

But Beth is eager to get back to the story of Butch. It begins in the early 1970s, when a cat belonging to one of her coworkers gave birth to a litter. Beth quickly offered to adopt two of the kittens, but not long after she brought them home, tragedy struck.

"I happened to have a litter of puppies at that time, and these silly kittens wouldn't stay out of the puppy pen. Either the puppies played them to death or they were eaten by coyotes or something," she says. "One morning I found them dead. I was just devastated."

Some weeks later, Beth ran into her coworker and learned from him that he was planning to take the last remaining kitten from that litter to the local humane society that very same day. "I'm too much of an animal lover to have let that happen," she proclaims. So instead of a trip to the pound, the lucky feline made its way out to her sprawling ranch—this time under the very watchful eye of his new owner.

Beth laughingly recalls that from the beginning, Butch was an unusual cat. "That kitten was so arrogant. He would even box the puppies' ears. He became best friends with all my dogs—especially my collie. But he was always getting himself in some kind of trouble— from accidents to ringworm. I think he lost eight of his nine lives before he was two years old."

The most serious trouble that Butch got himself into, however, was wandering from home and into the nearby foothills. "That was the time I really thought it was the end of him," she asserts.

It was a very cold weekend, and Beth and Jack were on their way to a dog show in Nebraska. Somewhere along the way, they discovered their mischievous cat hiding out in the back of their van.

"Well, rather than go all the way back to the ranch, we stopped in town about a half hour from home," she relates. "My father-in-law, Vincent, was visiting friends for dinner there. He was on his way up here to take care of the ranch while we were gone."

Butch was turned over to the care of Vincent, who promised to bring the mischievous cat back to the ranch. "But when my father-in-law got to the gate," she relates, "he got out of his truck and completely forgot that Butch was in the backseat. He left the truck door open, and Butch jumped out." When Vincent realized what had happened, he drove around looking for Butch, but he didn't have a clue as to where he was.

"We got home about noon on Monday," she recalls, "and there was a note for us from my father-in-law: 'Did you find the cat?' My heart sank. I immediately took off and started looking for him."

That weekend the temperature dropped to five below zero. "This was an outdoor cat, but when you're lost and hungry in this kind of weather, things can happen."

For nearly a week, Beth continued her fruitless search for her missing two-year-old cat. The only luck she had was that the weather turned slightly warmer. "I kept leaving food, but who knew who was eating it with all the other cats and dogs around," she recollects. Still, Beth refused to give up her search. "One trait I have is a lot of perseverance." She laughs.

By the end of the week, the weather had improved even further, so Beth decided to take a long walk with her collie in search of Butch. Of all the dogs back at the ranch, the collie was Butch's best friend. "I walked over to our mailbox, which is by the front gate, and called and called and waited," she relates. "I knew that too often people searching for missing animals call and then move on too quickly. The animals can't find them. I didn't want to make that mistake.

"Then I sat by my neighbors' barn and read my mail, hoping that I'd see him. I remember that every time I called Butch's name, the collie's ears would perk up and she would grow alert, as if she were trying to help me find him."

Discouraged by the lack of any response from Butch, Beth began the two-mile trek back to her ranch. For nearly an entire week, she had been praying for Butch's return, but so far there was no answer to her prayers.

Besides prayer, Beth says she employed a spiritual technique she had learned some years back. This method called for surrounding anyone who was in trouble—animal or human alike—with God's white light.

"From the very start of my search—and even when I was most discouraged and returning home—I kept picturing this spiritual white light surrounding Butch," she says. "It's the same aura you see surrounding Jesus' head in paintings of Him.

"I kept focusing on the thought that I would be successful in rescuing him. I was offering up prayers for him while I kept visualizing this light around him. As I walked slowly home, I kept calling Butch's name."

During her walk back home, Beth kept praying to God, "If it is meant to be, please help me find my kitten." Despite her prayers, she was not feeling at all hopeful that her missing cat was still alive. "By now, I figured that coyotes in our valley had surely eaten him," she confesses.

About a half mile back from the ranch's gate, all the frustration of the week finally caught up with Beth. "I just kind of sighed, and muttered, 'Oh, Butch, I'm never gonna find you.' "

It was then that her collie's ears perked up again. This time, however, Beth noticed that her dog seemed to be more intent than on previous occasions. "She really seemed to be listening to something. Well, I also started to listen carefully, and all of a sudden I heard this funny animal sound."

Beth's heart began beating with excitement. Was that sound possibly a distress call from Butch? Beth didn't know it at the time, but it was Butch trying to signal her. "He couldn't meow normally because of injuries to his lungs. All he could produce was a thin raspy sound—but I heard it!"

Even as she slowly crossed the rocky terrain, stopping every few feet to listen to that strange sound, Beth doubted that it was Butch—it was simply too great a distance for a cat's voice to travel.

"In fact, it seemed impossible that he could have heard me or I could have even heard him, because the distance between us was so far," she asserts. "He was clear across the valley over rocks and draws and bushes.

"This was rough mountain territory," she goes on, "and I doubt that even if I had been yelling at the top of my lungs, a person or a cat as far away as Butch was could have heard me."

But the closer Beth got to the sound, the more her

hope grew. She clambered down a steep bank and transversed a narrow valley. Amazingly, and much to her joy, up ahead was what looked like a cat. "There he was, perched on this tall boulder," she recalls. "I found him! I finally had found him!

"He was so dehydrated and weak, but he leaped down from the boulder and ran over to the collie and gave her what looked like a hug around the neck. And my collie was wagging her tail like crazy."

Although it was filled with happiness, Beth's heart broke when she saw the poor condition her cat was in. "Butch was thin and starved," she sadly recollects. "He had a dislocated jaw, so he couldn't even close his mouth to meow, which is why he was making those strange sounds. In fact, he didn't meow or purr for years after that, until his jaw healed. Also, his lungs couldn't function properly, and he had pneumonia."

The trip back to the ranch was nothing short of a nightmare. The injured cat was in such bad shape that Beth had a very difficult time carrying it. "I was fearful of holding Butch in my arms for too long or too tightly because his lungs were injured and he was having a difficult time breathing.

"It took us about three hours to get home. I would run with him in spurts for as long as he would let me hold him, but then he would struggle to breathe, so I had to put him down to rest."

Now, thinking back to that ordeal in the foothills of Colorado, Beth is still mystified by the circumstances surrounding the rescue. Why, for example, did the run-away cat respond to her forlorn sigh of discouragement but not earlier to the shouting of his name?

"I'll never really know for sure. All I did was sigh,

but he somehow heard that sigh. The dog never barked once, so there was no other noise."

Having been raised in a religious home and, later, an active participant with her college Methodist Youth Fellowship, Beth does have one spiritual explanation to offer: "Maybe when God heard that sigh, He knew I had reached my wit's end and that I was going home," she explains. "I think that sigh told God that I needed help. I had done all I could do, and now this cat's rescue was in His hands. And so He gave me the help I needed.

"However you try to explain it, it was a miracle in the foothills," she proclaims. "Just maybe Butch would have made it home by himself, but I honestly doubt it. Most of the time around here cats are picked off by coyotes. And he was very ill. He wasn't even able to eat because he had a broken jaw."

As a result of this experience, Beth advises anyone with a pet in trouble—whether sick, injured, or missing—to pray, never give up hope, stay in action, and surround their animal with Christ's white light. "Even if you don't believe in Jesus," she emphasizes, "concentrate your energy and visualize light around your pet, keeping it safe. It's an aura of protection."

She also encourages owners of missing pets to stay in action. "I don't believe that God just hands us anything," she declares. "You have to earn it, you have to get it, you have to want it bad enough to do something. We can't sit and wait for our prayers to be answered; we must be an active part of those prayers.

"And then He helps us. I certainly wouldn't have found Butch if I didn't continue looking for him. I made the effort along with my prayers, and as a result, Butch lived for eighteen happy and healthy years after that."

12 · A Saint to the Rescue?

DOES Saint Francis, the patron saint of animals, still work his healings on animals? Severen Koski, a volunteer animal rescue worker from Columbus, Ohio, certainly thinks he does, and says her tale proves it.

Severen recounts a time when she brought home five feral kittens and their mother, who were rescued from the streets of Columbus. The kittens were in such poor health that a local veterinarian saw little hope for their recovery.

As an ardent admirer of Saint Francis, Severen turned to the revered holy man for spiritual assistance. The result, she says, suggests that the patron saint of animals is still able to perform healing deeds. "It was St. Francis who gave these kittens the power and strength to survive," the twenty-three-year-old animal rescue worker avows. "If you pray, he will hear you and respond to your prayers."

. . .

For nearly four months, Severen played housemother to a feral black cat named Eclipse and her new litter of five kittens.

Eclipse had run loose for nearly four years before she and her new brood were finally captured in March 2000 by the Forgotten 4-Paws, a Columbus animal rescue organization staffed by volunteers such as Severen.

Severen describes Eclipse as a "beautiful jet-black cat with gorgeous green eyes." However, despite her good looks, this mother cat had already earned a reputation among rescue workers as a mean and vicious animal who disliked people.

That didn't dissuade Severen from bringing the cat and her new family home for temporary lodging. Severen says she is used to being around unruly animals, having been raised in a family that always had both well-behaved and not-so-well-behaved pets underfoot.

"Eclipse was terrified when I brought her and her babies home," Severen recollects. "She had a strong fear of people."

It was a particularly cold Ohio March, and Severen made sure her new lodgers had the warmest room in her house. "I put them in my bedroom, and I separated them from my other five cats so that Eclipse wouldn't get more upset than she already was."

Problems developed a few days later when the kittens began to suffer from bloody diarrhea. "That's a big concern when you have kittens," she explains, "because they can dehydrate so easily and then die. So we started taking the kittens to the vet.

"It was one vet visit after another," she continues. "One antibiotic after another. The kittens were now having loose, bloody stools for nearly three months.

We tested them for everything but couldn't find a cause. We even changed their diet and monitored them daily."

Despite their continued medical care, Severen says that the kittens showed no improvement. "In fact, their condition was deteriorating. They weren't as active as they should be. I spent most of my evenings rubbing tummies and filling their bodies with fluids from a syringe to prevent dehydration."

With matters worsening, Severen says she decided to bring the kittens to another veterinarian to see if he could do something. The result was the same. Severen was now beginning to feel desperate.

"I was going back and forth to the vet daily," she recollects. "I couldn't believe there was no improvement in their condition. They were getting weaker and weaker."

One night, with the medical options running out, Severen says she turned to prayer. It was not a difficult thing to do because religion, she declares, has always played an important role in her life.

"We were raised in the steel-mill towns of Steubenville and Toronto, Ohio," she says, "in a home where my father—who was Catholic—and mother—who was Methodist—were always talking about prayer, faith, and hope. We were always very open to different beliefs and religious practices."

One of her earliest memories is of listening to stories that her grandmother spun about Saint Francis and the animals. Those stories, she recalls, left a lasting impression on her. "I always loved St. Francis because there were always these pictures of him walking around the field with birds hovering over him while he talked to the animals. He loved animals and so did I.

I thought it was so neat that there was a patron saint of animals."

That evening, while praying for God to help the critically ill kittens, Severen reached for her Bible. When she opened it, stuck between the pages was a prayer card with a rendering of Saint Francis on it.

"I had attended a Catholic high school, and this Bible had been distributed to all the students back then," she says. "Even more ironically, I attended St. Francis Church. The prayer card was given to me by my grandmother, who had a local pastor bless it."

Although she can't be absolutely certain, Severen strongly believes that finding that prayer card was a sign from above. "I don't really know the answer for sure, but I do deeply feel that God had sent me Eclipse and her babies to care for," she attests.

"I had done everything I could to make these kittens feel better through veterinary medicine, and now I needed some other means to bring about a healing."

Removing the prayer card from her Bible, she sat down on the floor with the kittens that evening and uttered a heartfelt prayer to the patron saint of animals. In that prayer, Severen asked Saint Francis to guard the kittens and keep them from harm.

"I was praying for a speedy recovery, because I was also getting worn out running back and forth to the vet's office. I was cleaning the blood from their litter boxes, taking care of my other cats, and working full-time.

"I also prayed that if these kittens were to die, that Saint Francis should take them peacefully to God's arms. It was the first time in my life that I had prayed like that for animals."

Then another idea suddenly came to her mind. Severen decided to touch the noses of each of the kittens with the prayer card. "I let each one of them sniff it. Then I kind of rubbed the cards on their bellies and prayed some more for their recovery."

Next, she pasted the prayer card to the cardboard box where the five kittens slept at night. Then, after cleaning the litter box of bloody stools one last time, she fell into an exhausted sleep.

The following morning brought with it a miracle, she attests. "I went over to change the litter box, and I didn't see any blood. And the kittens' stools were no longer loose. I was shocked. I couldn't believe there was no blood in the box."

She laughingly recollects that the first thought that crossed her mind was that "maybe I'm losing it. After all, what were the odds of a saint answering someone's prayers? But after three months of bloody, loose stools, everything was suddenly normal."

Later that day, when she returned home from work, there was another pleasant surprise in store for her. "Not only had their stools improved, but the kittens were acting spunky. Within three or four days, everything was back to normal."

Astonished by this inexplicable turn of events, Severen called to report the good news to her mother. "I said, 'Mom, you won't believe this. The kittens are just fine.' I went on to tell her what I had done and all about my prayers and about the Saint Francis prayer card.

"So what do you think?" Severen asked her mother.

"I think it worked," her mother replied. Severen still laughs at the memory of that terse reply.

"My mother believes in miracles, so she didn't hesitate for one minute," she says. "Then I talked to one of the other volunteers—she's also a religious woman—and she believed it, too."

Today, all the kittens have been adopted into loving homes, Severen reports, and all are doing well. Eclipse, she adds, is still at home with her, but Severen says she has not given up hope that the mother cat will also someday be adopted.

"When she first came here she was wild. She would hiss and growl whenever I approached her or her kittens. She hated me. She didn't want me near her. She hated the fact that I held her babies. But I had to. I wanted them to get used to people.

"Now she's mellowed out," Severen continues. "She hops up on the couch with me and she lets me pet her. She'll even sometimes come up to me and demand that I pet her.

"She's become a loving cat. I think that someday she'll stop running and hiding from other people and let them pet her. Right now only me and my boyfriend can get close to her."

Reflecting upon her unusual experience, Severen says she has become Saint Francis's number-one fan in the Columbus area and, maybe, in the whole wide world.

That's why she wholeheartedly encourages anyone with a pet in distress to offer up a prayer to this animal-loving saint. "It's not like saying, 'Dear God, let me win the lottery,' she explains. "Whether you pray to Saint Francis or directly to God, you must really and truly believe that your cat will be healed by divine intervention.

"If you do so—if you pray from the heart the way I did—I think that Saint Francis will hear you and come to your pet's rescue."

13 ▪ An Old Dog, a New Gift of Health

WHEN Mikko, a fourteen-year-old black Lab with white whiskers, eagerly bounds to the door to greet arriving guests, Rose Amadeo is filled with delight.

And why shouldn't she be? After all, this is a dog who at one time was diagnosed with a serious liver and pancreatic infection and was not given much of a chance of survival by her veterinarian.

But Rose, a Vurnaby, British Columbia, resident who shares her home with three cats and a dog, was not quite ready to give up on the old dog yet. She added prayer and Reiki, an ancient Tibetan energy healing system, to Mikko's medical treatment, and believes those additions—especially prayer—helped to save the dog's life.

"The power of prayer is everything," Rose declares. "If you want to get that divine energy moving, then you have to pray. If you could only see what happened to Mikko, you would pray, too."

. . .

When the sun begins to rise over her home in the suburbs of Vancouver, and weather permitting, seventy-seven-year-old Rose Amadeo likes to stroll out to a woodsy park not far from her house with her old pal Mikko to celebrate nature's splendor.

For Rose, nature, cooking, and animals have always been the loves of her life—especially nature. "That was very big in our family," she relates. "My mother taught us that we had to know our trees and our birds and our animals. I remember her teaching me how to identify every bird just by the sound of it. That's why I love all creatures. God created all of that—nobody else could but God, and I love God."

Her love of nature was one of the reasons why, in 1972, Rose moved from her urban Ontario digs, where she was born and raised, to her present home outside of Vancouver. Her house is located on a secluded half acre of land which gives her an uninterrupted view of nature.

Rose says there are days—both in her own backyard and at a nearby park—when she can observe everything from woodpeckers at work and scavenging raccoons to an occasional coyote hunting for its next meal.

"There's even a bird sanctuary in that park," exclaims Rose, who is known locally as "the bird lady," because birds always seem to be flocking to her house. "I've got birds always flying all around my house, and geese walking around my yard," the good-humored bird lover laughs. "You feed them once and they'll come visit you.

"I love it," she continues. "I'm a very spiritual person and love everything that's living. I even talk to the trees, and I sometimes feel that they're talking back to me. They're very calming and comforting to me."

Rose has a good reason for appreciating God's handiwork, having twice in recent years experienced the benefits of it personally. The first time was ten years ago when she was successfully operated on for a brain tumor. And then, more recently, when Mikko fell ill and made a remarkable recovery.

"Both of these healings were miracles in my life," she declares with conviction. "There was a time when I couldn't even walk. But here I am, out of my wheelchair, looking after myself and doing everything on my own. And Mikko is perfectly fine. It's wonderful. So I count my blessings as well as Mikko's blessings every day."

Rose and Mikko have a long history, going back nearly fourteen years when she first rescued the Lab from a local animal shelter. "We had a malamute that died, and I wanted another dog. So my husband and I went down to the ASPCA. There were several little black puppies running around like crazy, and this little one came and jumped at my arm. I said, 'That one is mine.'

"And I've loved her from that day on. She's been a wonderful, perfect, angel dog. I've had animals all my life, but she's special. There's a certain connection between us that I can't even explain. She knows exactly what I want even before I ask her."

Rose adds that her affinity for animals dates back to her childhood. "I had animals around me since the day I was born," she declares. "There were cats and dogs and all kinds of animals. It's not home without a pet.

Even when I grew up and got married, there were always dogs and cats in my house."

Problems with Mikko began to develop several months ago. "She started dripping a bit," Rose says, "and so I took her to the Alta Vista Animal Hospital. They found she has Cushing's disease, a condition caused by a pituitary gland malfunction and she was given some medication. She started to come along fine."

Then, several weeks later, new symptoms developed. "She started dragging herself around the house," Rose recollects. "I said, 'Mikko, what's the matter? You never walk like that?' She was walking with her tail between her legs, her head down, and her eyes were funny.

"I thought I'd give her a day, and if she didn't improve, I'd take her back to the vet. When her condition didn't get any better, I had my son take her over to the doctor's office." The news her son received wasn't good.

"The vet told my son, 'Don't expect to be taking this dog home. She's old, she's losing her hearing, and she has cataracts.' Then he ran tests and found she had an infection in her liver and her pancreas. He gave Mikko some medication and placed her on an IV."

Rose was devastated by the veterinarian's diagnosis. "How can I explain what I felt when I heard that? I absolutely love that dog. I told my son to let the vet do what he can do for her, but I'm not going to let her suffer."

While Mikko was being treated at the animal hospital, Rose sought the help of other pet owners on various Internet prayer lines. "I E-mailed the situation to the Healapet Web site, where I knew that hundreds of animal lovers would begin praying for Mikko."

Next, she began praying on her own. Rose says she turned to prayer because it's a powerful healing tool, and one with which she has long been familiar. "I was brought up believing in God and angels," she explains.

"I wouldn't say I was brought up in a religious family in the sense that we were going to church all the time, but it was a very God-fearing family. God was always in our life. My mother always stressed that we had guardian angels. 'Ask for them and they'll be there', she used to say."

Rose, a Reiki healer, also transmitted healing energy to her ailing dog. When the sick dog returned home for what the veterinarian expected to be its final days, Rose spent hours "massaging, holding, and comforting her, because I loved that dog.

"I would do that maybe ten or eleven times a day," she relates. "At night, when I was saying my prayers, I would ask God to help her. And the first thing in the morning I would go outside of the house and also pray for her. What else could I do?"

Two days later, Rose believes she witnessed a remarkable example of divine intervention. "It just had to be," she says, "because Mikko started feeling just fine. I called the animal hospital and I think they were all surprised.

"And she's still absolutely fine," Rose declares. "She couldn't even walk before—she was lying there on death's doorstep—and now I take her out every morning and every night and she's perfectly normal. And this was a dog that just a few days before, the vet was ready to put down. Now she has a new lease on life."

Rose believes the miracle she witnessed was a combination of things—proper medical care, Reiki, and the most important ingredient of all, lots of prayer. "If it wasn't for me and all the people across the country praying for her, I don't think Mikko would have lived," she says. "The power of prayer is everything—it's everything," she emphasizes.

"If we couldn't talk to God and ask for His help, where would we be? You know, I had to raise six children, and I had to work besides. If He didn't help me, how would I ever have managed? I couldn't have. He's everything!"

Trying to put it all into perspective, Rose says that "it really doesn't matter how much medication an animal is given. If God believes it's time for an animal to go, that animal will die. In this case, God decided it wasn't Mikko's time yet. And I think all the prayers helped to convince Him to keep Mikko around.

"Every night I thank God for my healing from a brain tumor and for His healing of Mikko," she submits. "Get that energy flowing and keep in mind that it comes from the Divine."

14 · The Crackhouse Kitten

WHEN New York City police raided a crackhouse in Spanish Harlem, the last thing they expected to find in this den of iniquity was a black kitten acting a bit wild but otherwise in good health.

And the last thing that Patricia A. Leone, a playwright, documentary filmmaker, and the owner of a construction consulting firm, expected when she first saw Mykos at the humane society shelter, was that she would be bringing this former crackhouse kitten home—especially since the kitten didn't have the exact coloring that Patricia was searching for in a cat.

When, some days later after arriving at her home, Mykos fell seriously ill, Patricia first turned to conventional veterinary medicine. But the kitten failed to respond to such treatment, so Patricia took a different approach—one which she contends led to a miraculous recovery.

That experience has prompted the construction industry executive to pursue a dream—establishing the

nation's first holistic and spiritual healing center for
animals.

■   ■   ■

Seated in her chic Greenwich Village apartment over-
looking New York City's Hudson River, the diminutive, blond-haired fifty-year-old cradles Mykos—
named after the Greek Island of Mykonos, which she
fell in love with on a visit—in her arms as she talks
about the nine-and-a-half-year-old cat's obviously
charmed life.

Patricia is an energy-filled multitalented woman. In
addition to running the Dakota Consulting Corporation,
a firm that designs and builds commercial and residen-
tial spaces, she has also written and produced a play
about James Dean. Recently, she finished a documentary film.

Patricia wears yet another hat that she's proud of—
that of a spiritual healer. It's a talent she inherited from
her mother. "I grew up in Westchester in a household
where the Catholic religion was important," she explains. "My mother was a very spiritual woman who
did faith healings for many people. I think I inherited
that ability."

Her interest in healing has led Patricia to devote her
life to the study of many healing modalities, at the top
of the list of which she places prayer. "One of the most
powerful healing tools is prayer," she submits. "Sometimes medicine just doesn't work, but God always
does."

Another keen interest of hers is animals. "The neighborhood my family grew up in was a poor one, and
there were stray animals running around all the time,"

she says. "I remember my sister and I were always finding dogs and cats and bringing them home. My mother was also constantly saving animals and bringing them home. We had three dogs and a cat all the time I was growing up."

Even when she left New York to attend the University of Colorado, where she majored in prelaw, political science, and theater, Patricia continued her animal rescue work.

"Soon after I arrived there I found a dog in the park that I took in, and then any stray animal that came by my door. If they were hurt or needed medical attention, I would take care of them. Over the years, I've saved birds, squirrels—you name it."

When she returned to New York City in 1991, Patricia wanted to get a kitten as company for her fifteen-year-old cat, Ian. Ian was a jet-black cat, and being something of an aesthete, Patricia wanted a kitten of the same color.

"I went to the humane society shelter a couple of times," she recalls, "but nothing clicked. I also wanted a black cat because I think they're very intelligent and spiritual animals."

In September of that year, Patricia and a friend returned to the shelter to take another look. "There was a black kitten there who was about five weeks old. I picked him up and saw that he had a white spot on his tummy.

"And I said, 'No, what I'm really looking for is an all-black cat.' And so I put him back and left. Later, my friend said, 'You wanted a male, he's mostly black, and he's real cute. Why don't we go back and look at him again.' "

Patricia agreed to take a second look, and this time she had a change of heart. "I learned that he was found in a crackhouse by the police. He was very skittish and on the wild side, and to this day if I open aluminum foil or anything that he associates with what was going on back then, he'll run away."

When she heard the story of Mykos's rescue, her heart went out to the unfortunate cat. She plunked down a forty-five-dollar adoption fee and brought her new pet home.

"For about three or four days he was just like any other kitten, running around and being frisky," she recalls. "A few days later, he started to get very listless. I didn't think much about it. I kept an eye on him for a few days, and then he got worse. He became very ill."

Patricia called the humane society and says she got an answer that wasn't very humane. "They said, 'Just bring him back and we'll give you another kitten.' I said, 'Well, what are you going to do with him?' They said, 'Don't worry, just bring him back.'

"I just knew that if I brought Mykos back there, it would mean the end of his life. So I took him to my veterinarian, who diagnosed him with some kind of viral infection. He had a lot of tests, and he was hospitalized for a while," Patricia relates. "Although I had spent hundreds of dollars on medications, nothing was making much of a difference. He still was very sick. He wasn't getting any better."

Patricia continued to nurse Mykos following her veterinarian's instructions, but the kitten continued to grow weaker. It was then that she decided enough was enough, and turned to a more intuitive form of healing.

"He had had the best of medical attention, but he still wasn't getting any better," she offers. "Things weren't working for him. I'd been a believer in healing since I watched my mother healing people as a child, so I decided to try to do what I could.

"I had a pendulum which I'd used for answering health questions and for clearing energy, and I used that on Mykos," she explains. "I also did a lot of praying. Whatever type of healing I knew how to do, that's what I did on him.

"I always kept in my mind that God was with him and in him, and that Mykos would be taken care of. I really believed that and put a lot of energy into that conviction."

Patricia emphasizes that Mykos's recovery was not an overnight one. "It took two or three months, but he started to get on his feet again. And I believe to this day that prayer was the primary reason."

Was Patricia surprised at the result? Absolutely not, she declares. "I so much believe in God, and that God is the source of everything we need. I really think that God heard my prayers. I think the faith and love I gave Mykos when his medical treatment wasn't working is what saved his life."

Patricia adds that this wasn't the only time that Mykos responded to prayer. She relates that some years later the cat had a urinary infection that was so severe, her vet didn't think he was going to make it. "Once again I prayed and prayed that he would get through this—and he did."

Patricia says one of her dreams is to open a holistic wellness center for animals where spiritual treatment and alternative medicine can be combined with traditional medical care to help heal animals.

"I'd like to someday purchase a building and design it especially for animals and their well-being," she asserts. "It would be a natural healing center that would specialize in the treatment of sick and abandoned animals. I'd like to name the center after Mykos because of the healing miracles that took place in his life."

15 ▪ A Minister's "Small" Miracle

WHEN the Reverend Ruth Ellen Bates's beloved golden Labrador retriever, Johann Sebastian Bark, recently came down with a serious eye infection and medicine didn't work, the Wellsburg, West Virginia, Presbyterian minister, writer, and teacher feared that the dog might go blind.

Reverend Bates, who describes herself as an ardent admirer of Saint Francis of Assisi, the patron saint of animals, decided to try something which she had only done before with people—the laying on of hands.

That experiment resulted in what she likes to describe as a "small miracle," and has prompted her to give thought to expanding her healing ministry to one that includes animals as well as humans.

▪ ▪ ▪

Reverend Bates is an enthusiastic believer in the healing power of prayer. "I believe there's so much power in praying for healing," she asserts. "I also believe that *anyone* who is religious—and I don't just mean Christians—can effect healing through prayer. Most people I know don't realize the power they have to heal. Even for myself, right now, I'm feeling the tremendous effect of prayer on an illness I'm struggling with."

Her conviction about the healing power of prayer can be traced to her childhood in Pennsylvania and, later, West Virginia, where she grew up the daughter of a Presbyterian minister who spoke often to his family about the miraculous qualities of prayer.

"Both my parents were religious, and we always prayed together as a family," she says. "They not only read and talked about religion, but they also practiced it in their everyday lives."

Reverend Bates adds that her parents were "extremely generous people who helped the poor, immigrants—and even sponsored people from very poor areas of the world to come and live in the United States. Sometimes these people would live in our home."

Since she'd been raised in that kind of compassionate environment, it isn't surprising that this young woman would eventually enter the ministry. Reverend Bates agrees that for most of her life she has, indeed, always felt a calling to help anyone—human and animal—who is in trouble.

"It's always seemed natural for me to help people who were suffering," she attests. "If our family wasn't helping out people, we were always befriending runaway dogs and trying to find homes for them."

The diminutive minister who holds a doctor-of-divinity degree as well as a doctorate in creative writing, laughingly relates that although there were "always cats and fish around the house—and a few pet rodents—and although we were always saving dogs, we never had any dogs of our own."

Reverend Bates acknowledges that it may be to make up for that lack of canine company in her early life that over the years she has owned four golden Labrador retrievers.

Her latest canine companion, Johann Sebastian Bark, is a year-and-a-half-old, 110-pound golden Lab. "He's a gorgeous dog, but very mischievous." She grins. "I purchased him from a breeder and immediately fell in love with this affectionate and gregarious puppy. And even though he's a little over a year old, he still acts very much like a puppy."

But this past March, Johann suddenly developed medical problems. "A good friend of mine was watching the dog for a while because I was undergoing some medical treatment. When I went to pick Johann up, I thought at first that he had been attacked by another animal because he had scratches around his eyes."

When she returned home with her dog, his condition seemed to worsen. "His eyes were getting puffier and puffier, so I immediately started praying about it. I tried to find out from my friend the cause of it, but she said she hadn't even noticed that anything was wrong with the dog.

"All I knew was that Johann looked very tired, and he kept scratching his eyes. The next day, he woke up with all this puffiness and he kept scratching at his eyes."

Growing concerned, Reverend Bates worried that the retriever might seriously harm himself if he kept scratching at his eyes. That's when she decided to try something she had only done with people in the past—the laying on of hands.

"I feel a little funny talking about this, because it's not something that I'd ever done before," she says. "But still, there's something that happened that day, and it just shows how prayer can have a tremendous effect."

The immediate result of her experiment was that Johann began to relax. "I immediately noticed that he began to act differently. He's a big puppy and he never really settles down, but now he did. He seemed to like the warmth of my hands on him. There was something in the power of touching that calmed him down."

Afterward, she called her veterinarian, who prescribed a drug for the golden Labrador retriever. But that medication did little to alleviate Johann's discomfort.

"Now I was really scared about his eyes, because they looked so infected," she says. "I thought he would lose his eyesight or something. I kept calling my vet, but he was busy with surgery.

"I took Johann to the animal hospital, and the vet said he was pretty sure that Johann was suffering from some allergy."

Although the veterinarian prescribed different medications for Johann—including a shot of cortisone—the dog's condition did not improve. "So I kept praying for him and laying hands on him," she relates.

"Each time I laid my hands on Johann, I visualized that Saint Francis was touching him. I prayed, 'Jesus, touch this animal and heal the swelling of his eyes. Heal him of this particular allergy.' And I could tell that every time I touched him, he liked that. He settled down a little more."

One morning, Reverend Bates left the house for several hours to keep a medical appointment. When she returned, Johann looked much better—the puffiness around his eyes was less in evidence. "He also seemed much calmer," she recalls. "He wasn't scratching his eyes as often. I kept praying for him and praying for him, and pretty soon he wasn't scratching his eyes at all! This may not seem like a very dramatic miracle," she proclaims, "but I'm grateful for it nonetheless."

The clergywoman is convinced that without her prayers and the laying on of hands, Johann's condition might have worsened, because her dog was not responding to medical treatment.

This "small" miracle, as she modestly describes it, has prompted her to pursue more use of hands-on healing both with human members of her congregation and their pets.

"In the twenty years that I've been a minister, I've always tried to touch my parishioners in some way in my healing work," she explains, "but certainly not the way I've been doing lately.

"I've been doing huge amounts of reading about spiritual healing, and now I find myself praying more aggressively and trying to do more and more hands on healing.

"Its my own suffering from illness that has rekindled my interest in the power of God to heal and the ability of humans and animals to be used as instruments of God's healing," she declares. "And I'm now convinced that prayer and spiritual touch work not just for human beings but for animals as well."

Reverend Bates does not believe her conclusion goes against any church teachings. "We have great teachings on the spiritual healing of animals in both the Old and New Testaments," she explains.

One example she is fond of citing involves her favorite saint—Saint Francis of Assisi. "He had a ministry for animals, and was known for his love of animals," she proclaims. "He related to birds, and even tamed a wild wolf who was harming people."

The minister proclaims that if more people followed the venerable saint's example and expressed concern for the welfare of animals, "it would almost eliminate the need for animal shelters and putting strays to sleep. It would mean that every person who professes a belief in God would, indeed, also show compassion for the downtrodden animals."

Meanwhile, as a result of the "small" miracle which she experienced, Reverend Bates is now considering making a big change in her healing ministry. In addition to using hands-on healing for her human congregants, she wants to do more hands-on healing of animals.

"Just the other day, when I stopped to get something to eat, I told the waitress about what happened with Johann. And she asked me to help her with her dog, who was sick.

"God works in very mysterious ways," she exclaims, "and I think that as time progresses, this ministry is going to open up more to help animals. I think animals are going to be a much more important part of my ministry than I ever realized they would be."

16 . The Kancer Kat Bounces Back

(Editor's Note: In May 2001, a few weeks after this interview, Sam passed away from a related illness. Nancy's thoughts on her cat's passing follows this story.)

NANCY Dziedzic says her allergy to cats did not make her eager to have a furry critter scooting around the house, but when her roommate insisted that they get one, the freelance writer and editor reluctantly agreed to give it a try.

From the moment Nancy set foot in the animal rescue shelter and cuddled Sam in her arms, she decided that allergy or no allergy, this cat was going to check out of the pound and into her life.

Nancy didn't realize it at the time, but that friendship was going to dramatically change her life. Sam not only inspired her to move closer to God, but is the main reason why today, Nancy is busy with a new avocation—establishing her own local rescue organization to help feral cats.

. . .

If you can access the Internet and locate the Best
Friends website, you'll find on it a "Prayers, Healing,
and Support Forum" for pet owners. There, you'll discover a couple of messages from Nancy regarding her
longtime feline companion, Sam.

All the messages, you'll also notice, read the same:
KANCER KAT BOUNCES BACK WITH A VENGEANCE

In her message, Nancy gratefully proclaims that her
feisty feline is "doing so well, she doesn't have to go
back to the vet for a month." She also extends thanks
to members of the forum, who, in December of last
year, offered up prayers for Sam's recovery when the
cat was undergoing cancer surgery.

Nancy ends her message with this piece of advice:
"I just want to tell all of you who are right now de-
spairing over the illness of an animal that sometimes
there is hope where there seems to be none. Prayers
work, miracles happen. Keep believing."

It's a piece of advice that comes straight from her
heart. It also comes from a young woman who grew
up in a Roman Catholic household where formal religion was quite important.

"I remember as a child that we went to church every
Sunday," Nancy relates. "My mother had an especially
strong faith because she went through a whole lot in
her life. She always emphasized volunteerism and
helping people—she's a big believer in the more you
give the more you get."

That spirit of helping others seems to have rubbed
off on Nancy, who, when Sam was diagnosed with
cancer, devoted an incredible amount of time and effort

to assist the ailing feline. And she's still giving of her time to help other animals. Nowadays Nancy is organizing a local rescue group for feral cats.

Ironically, her life with Sam almost never came to be. Although Nancy grew up surrounded by various pets—she rattles off the names of birds, fish, rabbits, as well as a dog or two she has owned over the years—an allergy prevented her from ever owning cats.

So when, years later, her roommate suggested they adopt a cat, Nancy didn't think it was such a good idea. But her roommate wanted one very badly, so Nancy eventually agreed.

When she entered the Silver Lake Animal Rescue shelter, Nancy recollects that about the only thing on her mind was worry that her allergy would act up. "We were looking at the cats, and I was petting some of them, and I was feeling relieved because my allergy wasn't bothering me too much."

In one of the cages, Nancy spied a gray cat with white whiskers. "She looked like she'd been through a lot. I picked her up and held her, and she sort of sank into my arms. It almost sounded as if she were giving out a sigh of relief. It broke my heart."

Nancy immediately fell in love with Sam, who was then three or four years old. "She had these great green eyes, and this white trim with a sort of reversed raccoon look," Nancy laughingly recalls.

For Sam, meeting Nancy was a second stroke of good luck. Sam had recently been picked up on the street by city pound workers. She was two days away from being destroyed when the Silver Lakes Rescue Group adopted her and removed her from harm's way.

And now she was about to leave the shelter and take up family life.

When Sam finally settled in, she proved to be an exceptional house pet. "We brought her home and she was extremely lovable with us. I was hoping that Sam would bond more with Margaret, my roommate, because it really was her cat. I wanted them to have the primary relationship."

But it was Nancy with whom Sam established a special relationship. "After a couple of weeks, Margaret said to me, 'The cat is really attached to you in a strange way. When you go into your room and shut the door, Sam sits outside your door and stares at it for an hour at a time.'

"It just became clear that for whatever reason, Sam was mine. I really don't know what it was about me, because I really didn't overextend myself to her. She just wanted to be mine."

When the roommates separated, Nancy left Detroit for Royal Oak, Michigan, taking Sam with her. Problems developed last December when Nancy noticed that Sam's breath had turned foul. "My husband and I have another dog and a cat," she relates, "and one day our dog walked up to Sam.

"When Sam hissed at him, our dog looked startled and sneezed. Then he ran away. I thought, 'Sam's breath really has got to be bad for a dog to react like that.'"

She took the cat to her veterinarian's office to have Sam's teeth cleaned. Nancy certainly wasn't prepared for the phone call she received later that day. "The doctor said she found a lump under Sam's tongue, and wanted permission from me to remove it," Nancy relates.

The veterinarian went on to tell Nancy she was not certain why the lump had developed, but cautioned that cats had a tendency to develop mouth cancer. "I was hysterical," Nancy says. "That was the last thing in the world that I expected."

Nancy's voice quavers as she relives that moment. "Sure enough, about a week later, we got the pathology report, and yes, it was cancer. So we went to visit an animal cancer specialist, who recommended a second surgery for Sam. Around February, that's what we did."

It was the beginning of a series of surgeries for Sam. One operation seemed to follow another. At one point, surgeons had to remove Sam's tongue. From now on, the cat would have to be fed through a tube lodged in her side.

Despite all her medical care, Sam was faring poorly. "Her weight was dropping rapidly, and she kept tearing the feeding tube out of her side. The doctors weren't positive about her chances at all."

In addition to shedding countless tears for her suffering cat, Nancy turned to prayer. She had shied away from formalized religion after leaving home to attend college and graduate school, "but now I even started going to church again," she asserts. "I just knew that I couldn't stand by and watch her deteriorate. This cat was my soul mate. We'd been together for seven years."

Nancy had many sleepless nights worrying about Sam, but she remembers one night in particular when she prayed until the early hours of morning, asking God to give her direction.

"I said, 'God, you've got to tell me what to do about Sam. I just don't know what to do here. Please give me the wisdom. Send me a sign.' Later that morning, I went to visit her after her latest surgery and I was thinking, 'If I go visit her and she lets me know that she's ready to go, then we'll let her go. But if there's any sign that she's not ready to go, then I'm going to do everything I can to save this animal.' I just felt very strongly that she would let me know what she wanted me to do."

In addition to her own prayers, Nancy says that night she also turned to fellow pet lovers on the Internet for spiritual assistance. She E-mailed the Best Friends: Prayers, Healing & Support forum, asking animal owners to pray for Sam's recovery.

"I asked all of those people to send any good thoughts and prayers to Sam—anything," she recollects. "And they did! They're such amazing people on that website. They genuinely care."

The following morning, Nancy drove to the animal hospital, thinking that this might be the final time she would see her beloved cat.

That memory still brings tears to her eyes. "I walked into the animal hospital and the moment Sam saw me she started purring. She looked at me with those eyes and I could still see fire in them. She's always had a very fiery personality, and I could see that she was not ready to go."

But when Sam came home a few days later, matters got worse. "She promptly tore out her feeding tube, and we made a trip to the emergency room in the middle of the night. "The surgeons were worried that stomach acid had leaked into her abdominal cavity. If that had happened, they said, Sam would surely die.

"I was up all night frantic and praying to God not to take Sam. I was praying to God, saying, 'Please, please give me the strength to get through this.' "

The next day, the news was good. Not too much stomach acid had leaked into Sam's vital organs. "This time they gave her a different type of tube that was much harder to tear out," Nancy relates. "But that didn't stop her a week later from pulling it out. That meant another trip to the emergency room."

Nancy remembers that a day did not pass when she wasn't in the animal hospital's recovery room giving Sam love and encouragement. Despite the gravity of the situation, Nancy recollects laughing at Sam's antics during her convalescence.

"She was like a wild woman." Nancy chuckles. "She was all over the cage with a tube in her and bothering all the other animals. It was just so clear that she had all this energy and that she wasn't finished with her life yet. She had more to do on this earth."

Nancy is still amazed at how quickly Sam bounced back from all the surgery she underwent. "All I know is that all these doctors told us that they were doubtful Sam was going to make it. I really think it surprised them that she did.

"They worried that she couldn't last for more than six months on a tube diet and would eventually starve to death, but from day one she kept gaining weight. Even today, Sam's weight is up to a whopping nine point six pounds—almost as much as before the cancer.

"In fact, I was asked to cut back a little on her food intake," she adds laughingly. "She's also developing an impressive amount of mobility with what's left of her tongue. The doctors think she may even be able to feed herself some eventually."

Was prayer the something extra that helped Sam to survive? Nancy can only shrug at the mystery of it all. "I don't know if it was prayer or her own crotchety refusal to give up that saved her," she declares. "It's a complete mystery to me. All I know is that I prayed an awful lot, and she's here and as healthy as she can be, given her unusual circumstances."

It was some weeks after Sam was recuperating back home that Nancy received an unusual e-mail from someone on the Best Friends website. "This woman in Rochester Hills, Michigan, wrote that she was looking for help in rescuing feral cats.

"When I got that e-mail, I said to myself, 'This is a message to me from God. After all that I've been through with Sam, I've got to take some of His healing energy and use it to help other cats. So I'm working with some other women to start a nonprofit organization in Michigan to help feral cats."

As a cat owner whose ordeal revitalized her own spiritual life, Nancy urges other pet owners with sick animals to also turn to prayer in their time of need. She cautions, however, that behind the prayers there must be real faith.

"You really have to believe that there's something out there that's greater than yourself," she avows. "You also need to believe that there's something out there that has the potential to give you strength while you're going through your ordeal. It's like I said in my letter to the members of Best Friends. "Prayers work. Miracles happen. So keep believing."

■ ■ ■

Addendum: "I know that some people will wonder what is so miraculous about a cat dying in the end, but to me it is still amazing that we were able to spend so much time together after the veterinarians had virtually given up hope.

"Over the past seven years, Sam taught me all about loyalty, courage, and strength, and in her last months, those qualities were even stronger in her. She had the heart and soul of a hero, and her legacy will be long-lasting.

"I have had the privilege of meeting some of the most compassionate people in the world. They've become good friends and they've really helped me through this. I can't say enough about the Best Friends forum. What a beautiful bunch of people."

17 . The Cat That Came in from the Cold

FOR many years, Kathy Vyn-Glicken labeled herself "your typical skeptical journalist" when it came to spiritual matters. But an abandoned brown-and-yellow tabby named Serge changed her way of thinking.

It happened late one evening in 1998 when Serge, whom Kathy and her husband, Dan, had adopted, became suddenly ill. Unable to get emergency care for the cat, Kathy found herself relying on a source she was not much in contact with over the years.

It was a night of mysterious happenings, and when dawn broke Kathy no longer doubted that a power existed in the universe which she had denied for too many years. "After what I witnessed with Serge that night," she declares, "when it comes to the working of God, I've gone from being a skeptic to being a believer."

. . .

Kathy says she is not much surprised that Serge, a local feline "runaround" in the Chicago northwest-side neighborhood where she and Dan lived, should have had such a profound effect on her life.

"He was always kind of a special and unique cat," she laughingly says. "He was the neighborhood cat and very lovable. Serge's owners would let him out of the house, and all the neighbors took to him because he has a great personality. He loves people—he's like a dog—and he comes to you when you call him. He's also a great kisser."

Kathy, who fesses up to being a cat lover ever since she was a little girl, says that of all the cats who have purred their way through her life, Serge may very well be the most remarkable. Even her first one-on-one meeting with the local tabby was a bit unusual.

"Dan and I were living in a first-floor apartment in the Lakeview neighborhood," she recalls. "It was a crisp fall day and I opened the window. All of a sudden this cat jumped into my lap."

It wasn't exactly the best moment for her to make a new acquaintance. "I remember how busy I was that day, because I was on a deadline. But Serge just wouldn't get off my lap." It was the beginning of a new friendship for Kathy and her husband. "Serge would leave for a while, but then he'd always come back," she recollects. "We'd feed him and he would follow me around the house. Sometimes when I went shopping he would even follow me around the block."

Although Serge seemed to have plenty of time on his paws to wander about, he was not a stray. The footloose cat belonged to a family who had recently emigrated to Chicago from Eastern Europe.

"They had lots of pets, but they never seemed to take care of them," Kathy relates. "Even in the winter, they'd let these cats out of the house to wander around in the cold. The first time I saw Serge running around in the cold I said to myself, 'This poor cat. He's not meant to be running around in a super-cold Chicago winter.' "

Kathy is not exactly certain when Serge started to become a regular guest at their apartment. She believes it was sometime after his owners moved from the neighborhood, leaving him behind. "He'd hang out outside our door and cry for us to let him in," she recollects. "I guess he decided to adopt us, and pretty soon he became a permanent part of our household."

The new houseguest soon began to cease his wandering ways. "He didn't prowl around the neighborhood as much as he used to. He became an indoor cat. Once in a while we'd let him outside, but he was always anxious to be back with us."

It was sometime during the fall of 1998 that she and Dan noticed that something was amiss with Serge. "He kept throwing up," Kathy explains, "but we didn't think it was anything too serious—certainly nothing to go see a vet about right away, because cats sometimes have a tendency to do this."

A few days later, the tabby's condition suddenly grew worse. "Not only was he throwing up, but he was also crying as if in pain," she recollects. "Then he started to hide from us."

Kathy grew worried. "Having been around cats all my life, I knew that when an animal becomes seriously ill, it tends to hide from people. This was late at night and the animal hospital wouldn't be open until the morning. We were afraid that he might not make it through the night."

It was then that Kathy's husband made a suggestion which somewhat surprised her. "He said that maybe we should try prayer and chanting." Prayer was something that Kathy admits she had failed to pay much attention to over the years.

"I was skeptical when it came to the subject of prayer," she exclaims. "I was raised a Presbyterian, but about the only memory I have of church as a child growing up is that it was much more a social than a religious event for our family."

Although she had recently begun reading some Christian Science materials, Kathy says that "religion was still pretty meaningless and didn't make much sense to me. If I was interested in anything when I was growing up, it was psychic stuff."

Despite her reservations, Kathy agreed to give the spiritual approach a try. "We stayed up with Serge and prayed and chanted until I fell asleep from exhaustion," she recalls.

Throughout that long night, Kathy kept thinking about stories she had read in her Christian Science literature about people who had healed themselves and their pets through prayer.

"There was one story I remembered that had particularly interested me," she relates. "It was about a man who had healed his dog from cancer through prayer. I tried to keep all of that in my mind while I was chanting and praying with Dan."

That night was an unusual one in many respects. For example, dozens of neighborhood cats wailed throughout the night. "Let me tell you, this was really strange," Kathy asserts. "This has never happened since or before. All these cats were making these howling sounds. We could hear them clearly. Dan said that this noise went on even after I fell asleep."

Were the neighborhood cats holding a vigil for their sick companion? Kathy is not sure, but since that evening she has come to believe that "animals are very receptive to prayer. Maybe they were responding to the chants and prayers that Dan and I were doing."

When Kathy awoke the next morning, Dan could hardly restrain himself with the good news he had for her. "He said Serge wasn't throwing up and wasn't in any pain. I was just so happy to hear that.

"Here was a cat that looked and sounded like he was dying, and now he was perfectly healthy. I just sensed that this recovery was the result of our prayers and chanting—it was a miracle."

Later that day, Kathy brought Serge to the vet's office, where he diagnosed Serge as suffering from a severe thyroid condition. The vet also told Kathy he was surprised that the cat had made such a strong improvement in such a short amount of time.

"Serge is on medication now," Kathy says, "but there's never been any recurrence of the problem. I used to not believe much in the power of prayer, but now I do—and I've been reading more and more about it.

"From my readings, I now understand that God does not create disease, that He is good. And if you pray to Him, any negative condition can be changed. Disease has no power of its own. It doesn't have its own existence."

For anyone nursing an ill animal, Kathy believes it is important to turn to prayer. She further advises pet owners to get their spiritual lives in order before adversity strikes. "You just don't wait and become spiritual when you, your cat or dog gets sick," she asserts. "Work on your spiritual life starting now."

Kathy adds that for anyone who does not feel comfortable praying over an ill animal, one option is to take their sick pet to any Christian Science practitioner. "They'll be more than happy to pray for your animal's health."

18 . A Guide Dog's Owner Sees Hope in Prayer

Although blind since birth, Jane Lang has never had any problem seeing the positive effect prayer can have on both people and animals. Her most recent experience with the healing power of prayer involved her own guide dog, Matthew, who was diagnosed with a fatal form of cancer.

Jane, a church leader and public speaker, immediately turned to pet prayer groups, asking them to pray that Matthew not suffer any pain. She believes that she got more than she asked for.

Today, the retired Seeing Eye dog's cancer is in complete remission. Matthew is no longer actively guiding his master around. Instead, he is being guided along the road of recovery by a new Master in a most miraculous manner.

. . .

Jane fondly rattles off the names of the guide dogs she has owned since obtaining her first one in 1955, and for each, she has an interesting or amusing story to relate.

For example, there's Willie, who had a bit of a thieving nature. "Willie was a lovable golden retriever with one bad habit," she relates. "He liked to snatch things. He was the kind of dog who'd go into a store with me and try to leave with a stuffed animal.

"When the pastor of my church one day asked me to become a deacon, I was really happy and excited about that," she recalls. "Then he looked at Willie and said, 'Willie, you can be an assistant deacon, but this thievery must stop.' "

To this day, Jane still carries with her mementos of each one of her previous Seeing Eye dogs. "I carry either a pin I had when I got them or something else," she explains. "I still carry Willie's collar in my pocket. And on all their birthdays I buy flowers for them— whether they're alive or dead. You never forget a friend."

The mother of three grown children, Jane recalls that it was in 1992 at the Seeing Eye's international headquarters at Morristown, New Jersey, that she was introduced to Matthew, who was then two years old. Their meeting was a somewhat sad occasion, she recalls. "It was hard because he was going to replace Willie, who was still with me but too sick to work. Willie and I had been through a lot of stuff together."

Her new protector, however, quickly won her heart. "I remember that Matthew was the sweetest thing. When I brought him home, I was sitting on my bedroom floor petting his head. He had his chin on my lap. I said, 'Hey, boy, we've got a lot of miles to go together.' "

Jane describes Matthew as a "quiet and serious dog, who takes his responsibilities seriously." She says that's something she can relate to, dating back to the time when she was a youngster and attending the Perkins School for the Blind in Waterstown, New Jersey.

Her goal both then and now was the same; not to allow her visual impairment to prevent her from doing the things she wanted to do with her life. That's one of the reasons why today, Jane remains so active—as a church leader, public speaker, and avid sports fan who attends ball games whenever she can.

Her public speaking duties often take her before groups of school kids, businessmen, and senior citizens. "When I speak before these groups I talk about the work of the Seeing Eye organization," she explains. "I try to make the point that people are essentially all the same because everybody has some kind of handicap that they deal with in life."

If she's not delivering a talk on the subject of blindness, Jane can often be found at a baseball, hockey, or basketball game rooting her heart out for the home team. And when she's not talking sports, Jane has lots of stories to tell about dogs, because she has been surrounded by them for as long as she can remember. "When I was a little girl, my first dog's name was Pudgy," she recalls. "I wanted more dogs, but we lived in a small apartment in the city and there wasn't room for too many pets.

"I've always loved animals. I sometimes love them more than I do people. They're honest. They don't ask for anything back. They give you love with no strings attached. And you can always rely on a dog. I don't think you can with human beings."

Returning to her story of Matthew, Jane relates that things worked out well between her and the guide dog when she brought him home. "It was a great relationship—and it still is," she declares.

It was about two and a half years ago that Matthew became ill. "I was making a presentation before an AT&T group and demonstrating how Matthew would fetch things like my keys, but he couldn't do it."

Jane immediately suspected that Matthew was feeling sick and probably couldn't stand the taste of metal in his mouth. To make certain, she brought him to her veterinarian, who diagnosed Matthew as having a tumor.

After treatment from a veterinary oncologist, Matthew began to improve. Then new symptoms developed. "He was diagnosed as having lymphoma of the bone marrow," Jane says. "This was a different kind of cancer."

Matthew began undergoing another series of treatments, but the prognosis was not a good one. Because of the dog's age and his previous medical history, the odds were against his survival.

Jane, who grew up "loving religion," immediately turned to a Higher Source for help. As a deacon at the Presbyterian Church of Morris Plains, she placed Matthew's name on the church's prayer chain list—"and on every other prayer chain I could think of. People from all the churches I'm connected with and all my friends started to pray for him.

"Much to the surprise of the vet who was treating him, Matthew started to improve," she says. "It was an extraordinary recovery because lymphoma of the bone marrow is usually pretty serious business. It doesn't very often go into remission.

"But that's exactly what happened. And he's still doing okay. His cancer is in remission. He's eating well, and his blood work is fine. The vet can only shake his head in wonder."

Jane credits God and the many people who prayed for Matthew for this remarkable miracle. She says that a day hardly passes when she isn't praying for her dog's continued health.

"I ask God to please do the best for Matthew," she attests. "I don't always say, 'Keep him alive for me.' I do ask God to make my dog comfortable and to let me know what the right thing is for me to do for him."

Matthew, now retired, still lives with Jane, and a new guide dog, Laramie, has come into their home. "I told Laramie that we'll always work together, and that I'll never let him lose his dignity or suffer. I also promised that I'd never keep him alive just for my sake. If I feel that he wants to go, I will let him do so."

Jane is grateful that, to date, she has not had to keep that promise. "It's a hard promise to keep," she asserts. "You don't want to see your dog put down when the time comes. But you really have to be honest about whether or not you're keeping a dog alive just for your own selfish sake."

As she continues to pray and carefully monitor Matthew's health, Jane says she is making the most of every moment spent with her retired guide dog. "You know, if you make a commitment to a person or a dog, you keep that commitment.

"My mother taught me that. I made a commitment to take care of Matthew and keep him from suffering. And it is with God's help that I've been able to do so."

19 • A Dying Cat Sparks an Owner's Love

UNTIL a kitten named Mick-Bette came into her life in the late 1980s, Eileen Foley never related very well to animals. In fact, the Glasgow, Scotland, native says the only reason she agreed to adopt the kitten in the first place was because her boyfriend at the time urged her to.

Even after the part-Siamese kitten became part of her household, Eileen, an instructor of English as a Second Language at Florida's St. Petersburg College, remembers that for more than a year she carried on a lukewarm relationship with her feline houseguest.

That relationship changed dramatically, however, when the year-and-a-half-old cat was diagnosed with a fatal form of feline leukemia and given just a few weeks to live.

It was then that Eileen realized for the very first time just how attached she had become to this beautiful and feisty cat, and how much she loved it. In the days ahead, Eileen dedicated herself to saving Mick's life, and she turned to prayer to help her do so.

The result was not only a miraculous recovery for Mick, but an emotional healing for herself as well; Eileen says that for the first time in her life she learned how to love and nurture.

. . .

Eileen Foley candidly discloses that as a child, she never cared much for cats or dogs. "I was raised in a family which considered cats to be strange animals," she quips. "My family had some mongrel dogs who I wasn't crazy about either. I really never got along well with animals at all. I think I resented the fact that cats and dogs were sometimes treated better than people."

Today, Eileen has an entirely different perspective on the animal kingdom. She credits this change in attitude to Mick-Bette, a kitten she named after two of her favorite rock stars—Mick Jagger and Bette Midler.

"I believe animals are as receptive to God's love as people," she attests in her Scottish accent. "Mick taught me that, and I'm honored and thankful that this extraordinary soul shared my life for seventeen years and turned me into an animal lover."

That's quite some testimony coming from a woman who recalls a hot Florida day in 1982 when she tried to dissuade her boyfriend from bringing home a new kitten. "I had recently emigrated from Canada to the United States, and I met a guy in Florida who was a real animal lover. I didn't want any dogs or cats around because Florida is infested with fleas and I didn't want any part of that in my house.

"But my boyfriend's coworker owned a cat who just had a new litter of kittens. He said, 'Oh, please, come and look at them.' And finally, just to appease him, I agreed to do so."

Eileen says that despite her reservations, she was taken by Mick from the start. "She was a Siamese mix with this beautiful Siamese coloring and great blue eyes, and she was the firstborn of the litter."

Six weeks later, however, when her boyfriend brought Mick home, Eileen was less than pleased and cautioned him that it was going to be a temporary arrangement. "I said, 'We'll keep her for a few weeks and then you take her over to your mother's house.'"

Those plans changed, however, when the couple split up, and Eileen found herself with a permanent and not-really-wanted houseguest. "I never really bonded with her much," Eileen says. "She was a beautiful cat and I liked her and took care of her, but she was just kind of there. She lived her life and I lived mine."

In April of 1984, Eileen decided to go on vacation, leaving Mick in the care of a friend. When she returned home a week later, a shock awaited her. "I found Mick deathly sick," she recalls. "She was very close to death's door. She wouldn't eat, and she was so weak that she wasn't even able to walk."

Eileen says her friend at first didn't think much about Mick's decrease in appetite, attributing it to loneliness for her owner. "By the third day, she could tell that the cat was really sick and she took Mick to her vet. He told her that Mick had feline leukemia."

When Eileen learned the news, she was heartbroken. "It was at that point that I realized for the first time how much feeling I had for this cat," she says. "I knew I would really miss her if she died. I realized at that moment that the attachment between the two of us was really, really there."

Eileen rushed Mick over to her own veterinarian for a second opinion, but the diagnosis remained the same. "He said that Mick wasn't in any pain, and if I could get her to eat, she might live for a couple of weeks."

The vet also offered Eileen a glimmer of hope. "He said although this was a fatal disease, there was a slight chance that the leukemia could go into remission for a while, possibly giving Mick another couple of months of life."

Eileen loaded up on a variety of vitamin-laden foods, which she tried to entice Mick into eating without any success. "I laid out five or six saucers with different kinds of cat food," she recalls. "There was salmon, tuna—but she wouldn't take even a bite.

"The vet had also given me some Valium, saying that it often kicked in a cat's appetite. I even tried the trick of rubbing a little food on her nose to get her to eat. Nothing worked. She didn't even have the energy to lift her paw to wipe the food off her nose."

Eileen was devastated by Mick's condition. Not knowing what else to do, she turned to the one thing that had always sustained her. "When the food tricks didn't work, and the Valium didn't work, I just picked Mick up, took her into the bedroom, and I started praying.

"I was brought up Catholic," Eileen explains, "but by the time I reached my adolescence, I didn't want to have anything to do with organized religion. You might say I'm more spiritual rather than religious. But I've always prayed and I always believed in God. And that's what I did now."

She clutched Mick in her arms and asked God, "Please let this cat be with me a little bit longer because I really, really love her. I want to make her know that. I don't want her to die thinking that I never loved her."

Eileen went to bed that night certain that when she awoke in the morning Mick would be dead. "She was so sick that I didn't really have much hope for her.

"A couple of times during the night I woke up thinking she was dead because her breath seemed to go absolutely quiet. But then I would hear her breathing— her breath was so strained and raspy that it scared me."

When she awoke the following morning, Eileen feared her premonition had come true. "The bed was empty and I got real scared," she recalls. "I feared that she had somehow crawled away to die under the bed or something. I walked through the house calling her name, and there was no response. I couldn't find her.

"When I got to the kitchen, all the saucers of food I had left for her had been wiped clean." She laughs. "And then I saw her sitting in the living room, watching me look for her."

Eileen remembers that moment as if it happened yesterday. "I was just ecstatic and filled with hope," she proclaims. "I felt my prayers had been answered. But I still didn't think she was going to live long—I thought she'd have another couple of months to live and this was a temporary stay."

Eileen decided that with whatever amount of time she had with Mick, she would devote herself to proving her love for her furry friend. "I kind of dedicated myself to her," she declares. "I really spoiled her. I stayed with her as much as possible and let her know every way I could that I *did* love her."

The cat's wondrous recovery continued. Instead of growing weaker, Mick continued to gain weight and regain her strength. "A lot of her fur which had fallen out started to regrow and look good again. I called my vet and said, 'This cat can't be sick. She's gaining weight and is back to normal.' But his response was guarded."

Four months later, with Mick's health still on the upswing, Eileen brought the cat back to her veterinarian for another checkup. "The results came back negative," she relates. "The vet couldn't explain it. He just shook his head in disbelief."

Elated but wary of this too-good-to-be-true news, Eileen wanted a second opinion, and took Mick back to the animal hospital where the cat had originally been diagnosed with feline leukemia. "The results were the same, and they couldn't explain it either," she asserts.

"I truly, truly believe that Mick's recovery was a miracle. I know that feline leukemia blood tests are carefully conducted, with little margin for error, and that two different veterinarians had tested her and gotten the same results. But now she was just fine. She went on to live a happy and healthy life until she was seventeen years old."

To this day, Eileen believes that both she and Mick were blessed by the Creator. "Her recovery was a gift I'd been given by God," she declares earnestly. "Mick turned out to be the most effective teacher I've ever had. She taught me to really love and nurture, a feat that no human was able to accomplish. She became my longest commitment and purest love."

Based upon her own experience with Mick, Eileen has some advice to offer anyone who may have a dying cat on their hands. "Talk to your cat—that's what I did. Ask the cat to stay with you and tell the animal how much you need them and love them. And pray. Pray with all your heart and soul."

20 . A Dal Gets a Second Chance

SINCE 1999, Deborah Rickel, coordinator of the
Northeast Ohio Dalmatian Assistance League, has participated in the rescue of dozens of lost and abandoned
dalmatians as well as other dogs. But of all the wards
that have come into her care, the one that will always
stand out in her mind is a deaf dalmatian named
Chance.

When Chance developed a severe neurological disease and was given a slim chance of recovery, Deborah
decided to turn to the Greatest Healer of All for a second opinion. What resulted is the stuff that miracles
are made of. The dal who was not supposed to survive
found himself with a special blessing from God and a
second chance at life.

. . .

"I was the kid in the neighborhood who was always
bringing home the strays," Deborah says. "I've just always loved animals."

That desire to help animals in distress seems never to have left her. Even today, the forty-six-year-old computer programmer from Solon, Ohio, keeps busy doing animal rescue work.

When she's not at her full-time job, Deborah operates the Northeast Ohio Dalmatian Assistance League, a volunteer organization she started two years ago and describes as "a ministry." Even before forming the rescue group, she was keeping an eye on needy animals as a volunteer with a variety of other animal welfare groups.

A single mom with two grown kids, Deborah shares her house with seven abandoned dogs awaiting placement in foster homes as well as having three dalmatians of her own. It's not at all unusual for her phone to ring off the hook all hours of the day with people reporting animals who are in need of assistance.

That was the case one evening when she picked up the phone and took a chance on Chance. "I got a call from friends of a thirty-one-year-old guy who had found a job in California," she relates. "He had left his dalmatian with them, and had no intention of coming back for him. His friends said the dog was wonderful, but they couldn't keep him indefinitely."

Ordinarily, Deborah will not take in dogs who have been voluntarily surrendered by their owners because her organization is already overworked rescuing abandoned dogs. "I feel owners have a responsibility to find a home for their animals if they can't keep them," she asserts. "But for some reason, in this case I felt compelled to do something."

When Deborah went to pick the animal up, there was a surprise in store for her: Her new charge was deaf!

"I was really upset that the people who had the dog weren't straightforward with me about that," she says. "I probably wouldn't have taken him if I had known that, because our rescue can't afford to pay for special veterinary care. But I took him anyway."

Deborah admits that as much as she felt sorry for the deaf dal, at one point she considered putting Chance to sleep. One of the cardinal rules of Dal Savers—the national group under whose auspices she operates—is that deaf dals must be destroyed. Why?

"They go by the guidelines of the Dalmatian Club of America that stipulates that all deaf dals can be startled easily, and therefore they can possibly bite and become aggressive. So they need to be put to sleep."

Still, where there are rules there are always exceptions, and for Deborah, Chance was one of those exceptions. She smilingly recalls that there was no way that she could destroy this "handsome and sweet-natured animal. He turned out to be my most favorite rescue ever. I just fell in love with him."

Things quickly looked up for the abandoned dal. After spending some time at Deborah's home, Chance was adopted by a woman from Columbus, Ohio. Deborah thought that Chance's problems were finally over. Boy, was she wrong!

"This woman kept him for four months and then decided she didn't want him," Deborah recollects. "They just didn't bond. She returned him and claimed that he didn't sleep at night and kept her up all night."

But Chance's luck still continued to hold. "Another family said they were interested in adopting him. It was amazing—it happened right away," Deborah relates.

"This older woman called me and said that she had

a deaf daughter who was forty years old and slightly retarded. The daughter didn't work and was home all day. The woman said she wanted Chance to be a companion for her daughter. We sent Chance over and the two of them bonded perfectly. Chance was deaf and the daughter was deaf. I just knew in my heart that this home was perfect for him."

Again, the future looked rosy for the dalmatian but then tragedy suddenly struck. "Three days later—it was sometime during March—during a walk around the block, Chance collapsed," Deborah relates. "It was just instantaneous. He started shaking uncontrollably and just fell."

Adding to an already bad situation, Chance at the time was being walked by the woman's elderly mother. "She was a frail lady who had a heart condition, and she had to carry the dog home. When I heard that, I just felt terrible about what had happened."

Chance was rushed to the animal hospital and diagnosed as suffering from a condition known as myasthenia gravis, a serious and degenerative neuromuscular disease. "I loved this dog," Deborah declares. "When I got the report I was completely devastated. I think I spent more time over at their house with Chance than at my own. He couldn't walk. Every time he needed to go out of the house, someone had to carry him.

"The older woman couldn't handle it, and the daughter was slightly retarded and very childlike. She'd throw a fit and say that she couldn't do it. So I was over there almost every other night spending time with Chance and trying to help them out."

Despite all the turmoil, on her visits to the house

Deborah remembers being impressed by one thing—the great love that Chance showed for the deaf daughter. "He couldn't walk, but he could belly-crawl," she recalls. "And each time Michelle would leave the room, Chance would insist on belly-crawling after her. He didn't want to let Michelle out of his sight."

Meanwhile, the dog's condition seemed to be worsening. The veterinarian warned Deborah it was unlikely that Chance would survive his illness. "He said there was no cure for this condition. We were at a point when we didn't know if he would ever recover and walk again."

Deborah, who was raised in a Catholic household where no great emphasis was placed on religion and prayer, says something inside her prompted her to turn to spiritual assistance. "I went on the Internet and started searching for categories like pets and prayer, and that's when I found the Pet Prayer Line website," she says. "I was just thrilled to find that."

Deborah has kept a copy of the e-mail she sent to the prayer group's bulletin board. She reads from it:

> The vet doesn't know what is causing the paralysis and nothing is healing. I and his new family are just devastated and barely clinging to hope for a healing. Please pray and pray and pray for this special dalmatian that we love with all our hearts.

The response to that posting was overwhelming. "I got a lot of replies from complete strangers who said they'd be willing to pray for Chance. I also started praying for Chance every minute I could.

"I was constantly doing that. I don't pray formally

and I didn't set aside any special time. It could be
anytime day or night that I would pray for God to heal
this dog."

One week later, much to everyone's surprise and
Deborah's delight, there was a sudden and dramatic
improvement in the dal's condition. "Chance just
started walking—and I don't mean a gradual thing!
This wasn't just a little bit of walking. He started walking just all of a sudden."

Excited about this unexpected development, Deborah called the veterinarian to report the good news. His
reaction, Deborah recollects, was lukewarm. "He didn't
seem to react one way or another even though he had
given this dog such a negative prognosis."

Reflecting on Chance's miraculous recovery, Deborah is convinced that it was the prayers of hundreds of
people around the world that led to it. She adds that
the experience has played an important part in reviving
her own spiritual life. "I'm a more prayerful, and hopeful, and spiritual person now," she declares with conviction, "because what I saw at work here was nothing
less than the hand of God."

Deborah stays in touch with Chance and is happy to
report that the dal is still doing well. "He's back to his
old frisky self. He's doing so wonderfully. He's back
to being playful and loving. He's just a great dog."

21 • A Kitty's Double Miracle

CYNDI Wilson dubs her seven-month-old Maine coon kitten, Pashmina, "my miracle kitten." The Cleveland, Ohio, resident believes that the veterinarians who performed the delicate, lifesaving surgery on the critically ill kitten would certainly agree.

When Pashmina developed a rare feline bowel disorder just a few days after being spayed, the animal hospital's veterinary staff doubted the weakened kitten could survive a second surgery in so short a period of time. Complicating matters, the surgery was one which they usually performed on dogs.

It was then that Cyndi put out a spiritual S.O.S on the Internet, asking pet lovers everywhere to pray for the kitten's recovery.

Not only were hundreds of prayers sent her way, but generous pet owners also sent Cyndi financial assistance to help pay for the costly surgery. To this day, Cyndi avows that she will never forget this double miracle which saved her darling cat's life.

. . .

The story of La Princessa Bellissima Pashmina actually
begins with Cyndi's previous cat, Bullwinkle, a tabby
who died at age fifteen just before Christmas 2000.

"I really didn't want to replace my little bud-bud
Bullwinkle," she says, "but I wanted to honor his memory by loving another cat who needed a home and a
mommy of their own."

When Cyndi finally decided to get a replacement for
Bullwinkle, she set her heart on a cat with purebred
lines. "After a lifetime of owning cats that I had rescued from the shelter, I decided to fulfill my dream
and pursue a full-blooded Maine coon," she explains.
"I've always admired the Maine coon breed because I
like long-haired cats."

Cyndi and her husband, Leroy, began a round of
visits to local breeders as well as animal shelters. "I
thought maybe we'd find a breed close to the Maine
coon at one of the shelters or even a Maine coon that
had been abandoned, but there weren't any available."

When the couple read about a cat show in Toledo,
Ohio, they decided to attend. It was there that Cyndi
first laid eyes on Pashmina, and it was love at first
sight.

"We weren't in the exhibition hall for ten minutes
when I spotted this beautiful four-month-old-blue-and-
white-colored kitten," Cyndi recollects. "She was in the
first row of cats that we looked at, and I knew right
away that she was the one.

"She was sweet as can be and very snuggly, and
that's what I wanted. We took her home that Sunday,
and I decided to call her La Princessa Bellissima Pash-

mina." (Cyndi explains that this translates roughly as "The Princess of the Beautiful Fur.")

Cyndi can still recall how excited she was on that drive home with her new pet. "This was the cat of my dreams," she asserts. "She was totally different from any cat that I'd ever owned."

Things went well with the new addition to the household for about a week. "Then Pashmina started showing signs of being ill. She was listless and lethargic and was having problems with diarrhea."

Cyndi and her husband took the ailing kitten to the nearby Brecksville Animal Hospital, where the veterinarian immediately began to administer antibiotics and fluids.

"The next day, my vet called me and told me that whatever was wrong with Pashmina, it was beyond her scope of diagnostics and treatment. She said the kitten needed a specialist—and quickly—because her condition was worsening."

Cyndi was distraught, and in the midst of a raging blizzard, she raced over to the animal clinic. "I whisked over to one side of town to pick Pashmina up only to have to dash back to the other side in order to get her to the specialist before his clinic closed for the day—it was only open until noon."

The specialist ran a number of diagnostic tests on Pashmina. "The vet told us that little Pashmina had a condition called intussusception. It's caused when a section of the bowel telescopes over itself, and causes blockage of waste matter. It usually results in a bacterial infection that can be fatal."

Cyndi was also cautioned that if Pashmina wasn't operated on soon, she might die. The vet estimated that the bill for the surgery would be more than two thousand dollars.

None of this was good news for Cyndi and Larry. "I had just paid my local vet for spaying Pashmina, and now there was this added expense. And it had to be paid all at once. But I couldn't let my little princess die, so I told them to go ahead with the surgery."

There was another piece of disturbing news. The vet told Cyndi that this was an operation rarely performed on cats, because dogs usually suffered this condition. "They were going to perform an operation they were not very familiar with," she says, "and that worried me. They were planning to remove about ten inches of her intestines."

Cyndi was even more distraught. "My dream come true of owning a Maine coon had become a nightmare of worry and expense," she asserts.

While Cyndi was riding home through the still-raging snowstorm, for some unknown reason memories from childhood began to flood her mind. She remembered the prayers she used to say and the Catholic school nuns who told stories about miracles. "I was just fascinated by those stories of miracles," she recalls.

With those thoughts still in her mind, one of the first things Cyndi did upon arriving home was to E-mail messages to pet prayer groups on the Internet. She also called friends and family members and asked them to pray for Pashmina.

"I just knew that her chances of coming through this operation were about fifty-fifty," she offers. "Not only was she so tiny, but she had just been spayed less than two weeks ago and hadn't healed from that surgery yet.

"It was going to take a lot for her to get through

this, and I knew the key would be prayer. I had come from a family where prayer was important, so I knew its power. I also knew that God loves all His creations and that He would respond to prayers whether they were for a human being or an animal."

That night, Cyndi fell down on her knees and prayed to God. "I prayed, 'Let it be Your will to help Pashmina feel better and to give me strength during this ordeal.' " She also asked the Lord to guide the hands of the surgeons who were going to perform this delicate operation.

In the days to come, Cyndi says animal lovers around the world opened their hearts to Pashmina. The kitten's plight was posted on Internet sites such as the Pet Prayer Line and Cat Chat. Prayers on behalf of Pashima quickly began to arrive by e-mail.

Even more incredibly, members of the Cat Chat prayer group created a special website for the Maine coon kitty—picture and all—to help raise the much-needed funds for the surgery.

"Not only was Pashmina widely prayed for, but we were even able to get a little bit of financial help for her operation," Cyndi exclaims. "The breeder who sold us the kitten even chipped in to help us out financially."

For days after the surgery, Pashmina remained in critical condition. Gradually, her condition began to improve. "After several days of waiting and wondering whether she would recover, and only being able to visit her for brief periods of time at the clinic, Pashmina was able to come home," says Cyndi. "I was thrilled by this."

Reflecting back on her ordeal, Cyndi says she doubts

this story would have had a happy ending had it not been for God's help. "I truly believe that it was because of the prayers of so many—of people pulling together to pray for and to help Pashmina, a little Maine coon kitty that they had never seen—that she pulled through.

"It was prayer that put a lot of things into motion. It not only helped Pashmina to survive her surgery, but also created a warm feeling in us to know that there are so many people out there who are willing to help. It's something I will always be grateful for and never forget."

22 . An Ailing Dox Bounces Back

WHEN Snicky, a three-year-old dachshund, developed what doctors diagnosed as a crippling back ailment, Coleen Hartness of Lindenhurst, Illinois, worried that she could not afford the expensive surgery her pet required. Coleen decided that if she could not pay for the operation, she would put the animal to sleep rather than have it suffer and live out its life as a cripple.

Wrestling with this dilemma, Coleen decided to turn to prayer. What resulted, she says, was not money but something much more valuable—a miraculous healing.

Today, Snicky is living a pain-free life. "She has no back problem, no pain, and is on no medication," Coleen exclaims. "Our Snicky dog was touched by God. God made all creatures great and small, and if you ask for help for them, He's there."

• • •

Coleen can still recall a time when, as a young girl, she approached the minister of the evangelical church she attended and asked him to pray for her sick dog. The minister scoffed at her request, telling Coleen that "animals have no souls."

But even as a child, Coleen believed differently. She always had a strong affinity for animals, and sensed that there was much more to cats and dogs than just four paws, a tail, whiskers, and a cold nose.

"I believed and still believe that animals have souls," Coleen says with conviction. "Snicky knows right from wrong. She knows when she's been a bad girl. I believe that every animal has intelligence and a soul. Don't get me started about those people who say animals shouldn't be prayed for!"

Coleen just loves to talk about her "little Snicky dog." She says the six-month-old dachshund became part of her family after her daughter fell in love with the puppy.

"Whenever we went to the grocery store in town, we'd pass this pet shop, and my eight-year-old daughter, Kylie, would always look at this hot-dog-shaped puppy playing in the window and insist that we buy her. So my mother bought her."

The short-haired, red dachshund quickly became a beloved addition to the household. "For three years we enjoyed her as much as she enjoyed us. Everything was normal until about a year ago. Then, out of the blue, she started whining if you picked her up. I also noticed that she couldn't jump up on my leg when I'd approach her after coming home from work, and that's something she always used to do," Coleen continues. "This lasted for about four days, and things just seemed to be getting worse."

Coleen took Snicky to a nearby animal hospital

emergency room, where the doctor's prognosis was not a good one. "The vet ran his fingers down her back and said, 'I think there's something wrong on her back,'" she recalls. "Then he took X rays and they found that she had two pinched vertebrae."

The veterinarian told Coleen that back problems such as this one were common among dachshunds because of the long shape of their bodies. He prescribed muscle relaxers and anti-inflammatories for the ailing dog.

When three days passed and Snicky's condition did not improve, Coleen took the dog to her own vet to be reexamined. "He said, 'No, those medications aren't going to help her.' He put Snicky on an anti-inflammatory IV for forty-eight hours and told me that if the inflammation was not reduced in that amount of time, she was going to require surgery."

Coleen was quite upset by the news. "I said, 'How much will the surgery be?' We had just bought a new house, and there was very little money left in our savings, so I was worried about big cash expenditures. And he said, 'It'll be about thirty-six hundred dollars.'

"Of course I agreed to the surgery, with all intentions of begging this doctor for time payments, figuring he must have taken some Hippocratic oath and would not let my baby become crippled.

"I wrapped Snick in her bunny blanket and took off for our one-hour drive home. All the way I cried and prayed for help that the doctor would understand my financial situation and do the surgery without asking for payment all at once."

While driving home, Coleen made a difficult promise to herself. If the vet refused to perform the operation because she could not pay for it all at once, then she would put her dog to sleep.

"I couldn't stand seeing her drag herself over to me, looking up at me with those big brown eyes and asking for help," Coleen explains. "I couldn't let her suffer. I wouldn't let her live her life out as a helpless cripple. I cried and cried and wondered what I would tell my daughter, Kylie, if one morning Snicky was no longer around."

Coleen's worst fears materialized. Forty-eight hours had passed, and Snicky showed no improvement. When Coleen returned to the animal hospital, the veterinarian reaffirmed that the dachshund was going to need surgery very soon. He also ruled out payments for the operation.

Coleen decided to look around for someone who would charge less money for the operation. "We found another vet and took Snicky there for a second opinion," she relates.

"He also said that she was going to need spinal surgery. The price he quoted for the surgery was the same, and there would be no time payments. Again, my heart broke. I just couldn't afford it."

By now, Snicky was beginning to lose feeling in her hind legs and was dragging herself around the house. The dog was also being given morphine to ease its pain. "It wasn't easy for anyone in the family to watch this dog suffer," she says.

As Snicky continued to walk with difficulty, Coleen had yet another concern. The vet had warned her that if the dog lost feeling in its hind legs, it could mean a disc had ruptured and Snicky might spend the remainder of her life attached to a pet wheelchair device.

That Sunday, distraught at Snicky's deteriorating condition, Coleen decided to attend services at the First Christian Church of Gurney, Illinois. "Driving over to the church, my mind was racing with thoughts like, 'I'm going to have to put her down if she doesn't get better because I don't have the money. I can't even pay it out because they all want the money up front.' "

As she entered the church, Coleen flashed back to the last time she had appealed to a minister to pray for an ailing dog and the rebuff she had received. "But this was a different minister," she argued. "Even though I was feeling awkward, I decided I would ask him to pray for Snicky."

Coleen approached the pastor during a break in the service.

"What's wrong?" the minister asked, seeing the distraught look on her face.

"A little member of our family has a ruptured disc," Coleen replied. "We need prayer for her, because I don't have money for the surgery."

"Who is the prayer for?"

"It's for my dog, Snicky."

Coleen braced herself for another sermon on soulless animals. Instead, she was greeted by a pleasant surprise. "A big smile broke out on the minister's face," she recollects. "He said, 'Oh, I've never been asked to pray for an animal before. Okay, she needs it and she's a part of your family, so we're going to pray for her.' "

When the minister returned to the pulpit to announce the day's prayer requests, among the names mentioned was that of the ailing three-year-old dachshund. "She stayed on the prayer chain there for weeks." Coleen grins.

Coleen recalls that later that week she received a phone call from the minister. "He said, 'I'm so glad you had me pray for Snicky. I've had families coming up to me and thanking me for mentioning an animal. They were always too embarrassed to ask for prayer when their pets were ill.' "

The time was quickly arriving for Coleen to make a decision about Snicky's surgery. Still undecided, she began one evening to search the Internet for pet wheelchairs.

"That's when I found the website for the Pet Prayer Line," she says. "So I put her on their prayer list, knowing that hundreds of pet owners around the world would be praying for Snicky."

Meanwhile, Coleen did what she could to ease her dog's suffering. "I would place my hands on her back and pray each time Snicky was having a bad day. I'd pray, 'Please, God, I don't want to put this dog down. Help me find a way to get the money for the surgery, or heal her.' "

There are times when a miracle can occur swiftly, says Coleen, and this was one of them. "It happened just after Thanksgiving," she jubilantly relates. "I came home from work one day about two weeks after her diagnosis, and Snicky's back legs were beginning to move a lot better.

"She stopped whimpering and she wouldn't hesitate climbing up the stairs. I no longer had to give her any pain medication. She was getting better and better."

Right before her eyes, Coleen was witnessing a miracle unfold. Members of her family were equally amazed.

One of the first things Coleen did was call the An-

tioch Animal Hospital, where Snicky had been scheduled for surgery. "I told the vet, 'She's moving around
like there's nothing wrong. She's not hurting anymore
and I can pick her up. She's jumping up on the couch
and standing up to look out the window.' "

She remembers a long pause on the other end of the
line before the vet responded. "Well," he said, "I have
never seen a doxie recover without going through surgery. Bring her in and let me take a look at her."

Coleen returned to the animal hospital with Snicky.
"She ran around the room and jumped up in a chair,
which she hadn't done in over three weeks. I just stood
there with my mouth open. The doctor said, 'It doesn't
look like she needs surgery to me.' "

That very same day, Coleen sent a grateful E-mail
to the Pet Prayer Line. It read:

> I asked for prayers for Snicky, my three-year-old
> doxie with a back problem. Thank you all for the
> prayers. God has given Snicky a miracle. We
> don't know how, but she's back to normal. No
> pain or medication. Thanks to you and God.

To this day, Coleen remains grateful. "I just don't
know what to say. I just thank the Lord for this miracle. There was just no way I could get the money for
Snicky's surgery, and He provided me with this miracle. I attribute it all to prayer."

23 . The Run, Run Runaway

WHEN Sebastian got spooked and decided to bolt from home, the dalmatian touched off a search that involved nearly the entire city of Sheboygan, Wisconsin.

While looking for the runaway, Christine Bishofberger, founder of a southeastern Wisconsin dalmatian rescue group, found herself alone in the woods. It was there that something remarkable happened which Christine says taught her an important lesson about surrendering to God.

Since that day, Christine, who for many years struggled with her faith, has paid much closer attention to her spiritual life. She says it took a runaway dog to help draw her closer to God.

. . .

Religion never played much of a role in her upbringing, Christine attests. About the only memory she has of her religious life as a child is going to church on Easter.

Christine says she began to regain an interest in religion about fifteen years ago, a time when she was struggling to control her alcohol addiction. "It was a pretty deep problem," she asserts, "and I did everything you're supposed to do to work through it—Alcoholics Anonymous, psychotherapy, you name it."

Nothing, however, seemed to work. Things might have gotten worse had it not been for her husband, Larry, who was raised religiously but had also turned his back on religion over the years. At the time he was beginning to touch base with his religious roots and was encouraging his wife to do the same.

"He started to reestablish himself with the church," Christine recalls, "and it was a huge source of conflict for me at first. He was clearly changing his direction in life, and turning into somebody I didn't know. We both had not been religious people."

Meanwhile, Christine's drinking problem threatened to disrupt both her career and her relationship. She desperately wanted to change her alcoholic lifestyle, but she could not find the strength to do so. "There was nothing more I could do to help myself—I had tried everything." She sighs, remembering those difficult days.

Although she was still resistant to her husband's spiritual prodding, Christine is convinced that on some unconscious level it began to take hold, and she is grateful to God for that.

There was one particular day that Christine still can recall very clearly—one she considers to have been a turning point in her life. "I remember I was at work, and I was in total despair. I walked into the bathroom, sat down in a stall, and prayed. I said, 'God, if you're real, take this desire to drink away.'

"It was an interesting choice of words for me— something completely out of character," she asserts. " 'Take this desire from me' was not the kind of language I would ordinarily use. The phrase sounded spiritual, and I had no idea where these words came from."

After uttering that prayer, much to her amazement Christine was engulfed by a sense of tranquillity. "The result of that prayer was so profound," she exclaims, "that from the moment I left that bathroom I knew that I was a different person. And most incredibly, since that day I haven't had a drink or the desire to drink."

While that miraculous moment more than fifteen years ago may have started Christine on her walk with God, it would take an encounter with a shy runaway dalmatian by the name of Sebastian to help her pick up the pace.

Sabastian is also the reason why today, Christine devotes much of her time to rescuing abandoned, abused, lost, or stolen dalmatians. Her desire to help animals, however, can be traced back to her childhood.

She recalls growing up "about three-quarters of a mile from a flea market, where I could purchase animals cheaply or for free—especially at the end of the day. So, as a youngster, I was always bringing home animals—everything from guinea pigs to dogs and cats. We had a menagerie in our house," she laughingly relates.

"My parents were very lenient in letting me bring all those animals home. At one point, I even brought home a horse, and that's where my parents drew the line. I eventually had to return it.

"There was even a time when I brought home two mice. My mom was a little concerned, but I reassured her that they were both boys. Well . . . they weren't."

It was in April of 1994, shortly after her marriage, that Christine decided to purchase her first dalmatian puppy, and soon after she became involved with a local animal shelter. "Working there, I used to see abandoned dalmatians coming into the shelter, and I was sickened by some of the things I saw. People did horrible things to these animals. Then I got involved with a national dalmatian rescue organization."

One day, Christine decided to establish her own local rescue group. With a partner who was doing similar dal rescue work in nearby southern Illinois, she formed a regional Dal Savers organization for southeastern Wisconsin.

One afternoon, Christine received a phone call that broke her heart. Sebastian, a shy and timid dalmatian she had helped to place in a foster home in nearby Sheboygan, Wisconsin, had bolted and fled.

Christine had a special affection for this tall, lanky dog, who had been abandoned by its owners. "He was five and a half years old at the time he came into the shelter, and although I couldn't prove it, I suspect he had probably been abused. He was gentle, beautiful, and incredibly shy."

She learned that the dog had run away because his new owner inadvertently did something to frighten him. "The young woman who adopted him wanted to replace his collar with another," Christine explains. "We didn't know that she used a spike collar for her pets—that's one with prongs which slightly pinch a dog's neck. It's less damaging than a choke collar, but some dogs don't like the look of it.

"All it took was one look at this new collar with its prongs and Sebastian freaked. He bolted from the house. Then his new owner made her next critical error. She didn't call anybody for twenty-seven hours. And those are crucial hours—just like when children are missing."

Christine surmises that Sebastian's owner was probably very upset, angry at herself, and embarrassed, which is why she didn't call right away. "She thought she could find Sebastian by herself. She posted notices, made phone calls, but all to no avail."

The following day, however, the woman's efforts did pay off. She received a phone call that Sebastian had been spotted. "Then, unfortunately, she made another mistake," Christine explains. "She approached the dog with the same collar in her hands. Sebastian panicked and bolted again, but this time he expanded his territory."

Now realizing she might never find her dog, the woman finally called Dal Savers for help. "I got the message about eight o'clock on a Monday night," Christine recalls. "I immediately packed some clothes and headed out to Sheboygan. I told Larry that I expected to be there only overnight."

That was, indeed, optimistic thinking. "I never anticipated that the search for Sebastian would last a week. I got up there, checked into a hotel, and that became home base for the search.

"Because of my newfound interest in religion, I had already decided that I would be sensitive to God's directions, and that He would help me find the dog," she recalls. "I had to rely on Him, because I was a complete stranger in the area and didn't have a sense of where to go. So from the very beginning this search had a spiritual component."

Christine began her search for the runaway by driving around locations where Sebastian had been seen. After fruitless hours of searching, she realized that she needed more help. Soon, she was joined by volunteers from other regional dalmatian rescue groups.

The hunt for Sebastian was an extensive one. "We placed ads in the local newspaper, put up posters, and at times found ourselves searching for twenty-four hours straight without sleep. We even established a hot line at Sebastian's home. We got numerous tips as to where the dog had been seen."

Memories of that dog hunt bring a smile to her face. "It was like a military operation." She laughs. "We had a small army of people in Sheboygan looking for him. We even had train engineers and garbage collectors on the alert.

"We knew Sebastian was hungry and would be foraging for food, so the entire city of Sheboygan had their eyes open for him. Unfortunately, the dog was freaking out because everyone seemed to be after him."

Christine now worried that the dal would grow weary of being chased and flee deep into the woods. "There was a huge forest area nearby, and that was very frightening to us," she says. "If we scared him and pushed him out further into those woods, he was going to be lost forever."

For nearly a week, all attempts at capturing the elusive runaway failed. The frightened animal ignored dog traps, fled at the slightest approach of humans, and sometimes dropped out of sight altogether.

But throughout this ordeal, Christine always had a sense that God would eventually lead her to the runaway. "I would fall down on my knees and say, 'Please, God, I need your help. If you don't help me, Sebastian is going to die. It's winter, it's cold, and he's going to freeze to death.' "

Several more days passed and Sebastian was still on the loose. Then Christine remembered something her mother had once told her as a child. "She said if I ever got lost in a store, I should stay put. She said if you stayed in one place, you were more apt to be found."

Christine decided to heed that advice. Instead of hunting Sebastian, the rescue team would now stake out various positions and simply wait to see if the dalmatian showed up. "We knew some locations he would occasionally return to, so we decided to sit still, wait, and see what happened."

Implementing this strategy was not easy, as she was an action-oriented person when it came to her rescue work. Still, she decided to give this new strategy a try.

She remembers walking into a wooded area where the dal had been previously seen. From the moment she entered the woods, Christine felt that there was an almost magical quality to the place.

"There I was in this snow-covered forest, feeling the silence and tranquillity. It was perfect. It was also the perfect place to commune with God."

Christine did something which she had only recently begun to do again—she prayed. What happened next is something the animal rescuer says she will never forget. "I was given the word of God there," she avows with a note of awe in her voice. "I clearly heard the words, 'He will be delivered to you.' "

She also received a strong impression that God wanted her to continue waiting for the dog rather than pursuing it. When the impression finally faded, Christine sat there with a sense of stunned wonder.

"It was this incredibly awesome spiritual moment," she exclaims. "I watched all this activity in the silent woods—the birds, the chipmunks, other small animals—and I had such a reverence toward the magnitude of God and His creations.

"Most of all, I had a feeling of reassurance that this situation with Sebastian was not out of control—that God was in charge. As this peace and confidence washed over me, I thought what I needed to do was surrender and let God be God. After all, I had received His word that Sebastian would be delivered to me."

Then the old doubting Thomas side of Christine kicked in. Despite everything that her soul encouraged her to do, she failed to heed it. After all, it was in her nature and training to be active in search of a missing animal, and just sitting there certainly would not do.

"I just couldn't stay in one place and wait for Sebastian to come to me," she admits ruefully. "I couldn't obey that advice. Instead I continued chasing after the dog. I left the woods and put a new plan together that involved thirty-six volunteers from rescue groups statewide."

At the height of the operation, Christine received a phone call from her husband, Larry, who said he missed her and wanted her to come back home. It was a difficult decision for her to make, but Christine ultimately decided to return home.

"I cried the entire drive back," she recalls. "I was sobbing because I hadn't found Sebastian even though God's words of reassurance kept rolling around in my mind. I felt I had abandoned my search."

But in her grief she discovered something else. "I now acknowledged my helplessness in this situation," she attests. "It was like a final act of surrender. I did what I should've done earlier—I turned the whole situation over to God."

Christine is convinced that the moment she did so, miles away a miracle occurred. "I got home late Sunday night, and ten o'clock the next morning my phone rang. Sebastian had been found. He had suddenly stopped running and let himself be captured. He was tired and hungry, but he was on his way back to his home."

The phone call both elated and depressed her. "I had the sense that my inability to surrender to God was the obstacle to a faster rescue," Christine submits. "I felt if I had simply surrendered to God when He spoke to me in the woods and had heeded His words, Sebastian would have been delivered to us more quickly."

While Christine acknowledges that she will never be certain about any of this, there is one thing she is quite sure of—the importance of surrendering to a Higher Power. "I haven't been the same person since then," she offers. "For me, that episode was a lesson in obedience, a lesson about trust. I can't say that I'm one hundred percent obedient and trusting in God today, but when I'm not, I remember what happened that day in the woods.

"And what happened was simply awesome. Now I no longer feel I have to do something because I need to. I simply ask what God wants me to do. I surrender to Him."

24 . Jesus and the Frightened Kitten

FORMER opera singer Shirley Winston was concerned when Sheba's Shadow, one of five feral kittens she had brought to the veterinarian to be spayed, became frightened after her operation and hid from the animal hospital's staff. But Shirley was careful not to become alarmed and show fear. After all, fear is a negative emotion which does more harm than good, says the Virginia Beach, Virginia, resident. "If you feel fear, you broadcast fear, and that wouldn't have helped Sheba or anyone."

Instead, Shirley relied on silent prayer, sending peaceful thoughts to the agitated kitten. She also visualized Sheba's emergence from her hiding place. The result surprised most of the staff at the animal hospital, but not Shirley. Prayer, she emphasizes, can reach into all the darkest corners—even one where a frightened little black kitten is hiding.

. . .

Shirley Winston recalls that both music and prayer had filled her childhood days. The retired opera and Broadway stage star laughingly recollects that her mother—a Baptist—and her father—a Methodist—both taught Sunday school, but at different churches. However, Shirley was not much interested in traditional religion.

"They were very orthodox, but I was the one who, at about age fourteen, became interested in learning more about religion than just what the Bible teaches," she declares in a drawl that betrays her Southern roots. "I remember that I was taking voice lessons at the time with two women," she continues. "One was a Theosophist and the other was a Rosicrucian. They would tell me about reincarnation, karma—all these things."

It was those two women who were most responsible for her lifelong interest in metaphysics, which eventually led her to study the teachings of famed psychic Edgar Cayce. Today, Shirley writes and lectures internationally on behalf of the Association for Research and Enlightenment more commonly known as the Edgar Cayce Society.

Besides her strong interest in metaphysics and love of music, Shirley says she's always had an affinity for animals—especially dogs. The problem was, she notes, that as a young girl growing up in Alabama and Washington, D.C., she was not allowed to own one. Her family was constantly on the move because her father was in charge of the U.S. government's Soil Conservation Service, first organized in 1934 by President Roosevelt. That mobile lifestyle precluded dog ownership.

"We moved so often that I never finished a year in one place until I was in high school," she remembers.

"So I wasn't allowed to have a dog because my father didn't believe it was right for people who moved so much to own one."

Shirley's dream of owning a dog finally came true years later, on the day before she made her debut as an opera singer at Boston's opera house. "My teacher wanted to give me a present and asked me what I wanted. I said, 'I want a dog.' So I got two or three dog books and decided on a sheltie. After all those years, I finally brought a tiny puppy home."

That operatic debut led Shirley to a successful twenty-year opera and Broadway stage career that included international tours with the New York City Opera Company and the Metropolitan Opera, and lead roles in musicals such as *Oklahoma*! and *My Fair Lady*.

Her metaphysical interests, meanwhile, led her to a lasting friendship with Hugh Lynn Cayce, the son of the famous psychic. It was Cayce who convinced the psychically gifted singer to move to Virginia Beach, where he was then building the Association for Research and Enlightenment Center.

"That was thirty-two years ago," she recollects. "I was living in Greensboro, North Carolina, at the time. The one thing I remember most about Lynn is that he had a dominant personality and nobody could say no to him."

Shirley soon relocated to Virginia Beach, moving into a house on two acres of land which abutted a woodsy area next to a golf course. There, raccoons and other small animals were often regular visitors in her backyard.

Over the years, one of her most interesting visitors

turned out to be a family of cats who showed up in her backyard. "I had a neighbor who had a female cat—her name was Sheba—who she let run wild," Shirley explains. "And I would often see this white mother cat and her kittens going through my back garden. She had two little black kittens who always walked side by side with her, and one—a little black female—reminded me of a shadow. That's why I named her Sheba's Shadow."

Shirley began feeding the wandering felines, and soon they were regular houseguests at mealtime. "This mother cat kept on having kittens, and I finally decided that I had to do something about this—she was having two litters a year."

It was in February of that year that Shirley was finally able to gather the brood and bring them to the animal hospital for their rabies shots and to be altered. "I had two cats in each cage—there were six cats altogether," she recollects.

Several hours later, Shirley received a call from a worker at the animal hospital who apologetically explained that one of the kittens had bolted and hid when the holding cages were opened.

"I was told that the kitten was hiding in a corner behind rows of animal cages that were so heavy and full of other animals that they could not be moved easily. The kitten refused to come out. I asked, 'Which one?' and he told me, 'It's a little black cat.' It was Sheba's Shadow."

Although Shirley was concerned over Sheba's plight, she tried not to transmit any thoughts of fear. "I knew these cats were very scared being there in the first place, and I didn't want Sheba subjected to any more stress," she states. "Animals can easily pick up human emotions." Instead Shirley began praying for the frightened kitten. "I think of my cats as my friends, and I wanted to do something to soothe her. I was praying for her—and myself—not to be afraid."

After saying her own prayer, Shirley picked up the phone and called Meredith Ann Puryear, the Association of Research and Enlightenment's prayer services coordinator. "She's very good at prayer," Shirley declares. "And I said to her, 'I'm having a problem with Sheba's Shadow. She's gotten out and hidden.' And Meredith said she would pray for her, too."

Meredith recalls that phone call. "I told Shirley I would do what I could," she relates. "When I put the phone down, I asked in prayer what I could do. The first thought was that I project myself into the room, calm the animal, and coax her out. Then, immediately, it came to me that I should ask Jesus to go, because His very presence would calm all the animals, and Sheba would come to Him for comfort and healing."

Meredith recollects entering a deep state of meditation, thanking Jesus for His presence at the animal hospital. "I just sensed that all was well and proceeded with my meditation."

Meanwhile, a few miles away, Shirley was doing pretty much the same thing. "Prayer is the first thing I do when there's a problem to deal with," she asserts. "I have to get myself under control and drop any thoughts of being anxious over some situation. As long as there is any anxiety or fear in me, the only thing I'm going to be able to project to anybody is anxiety or fear. So when I pray, it's not really so much praying for anything to happen, it's about getting me out of the way of things, staying peaceful, and letting the Divine order function.

"When my mind is clear and I'm not worried about anything else, then I know that almost anything can be accomplished. Prayer helps me do that. It keeps me from struggling and worrying and being fearful. Then everything falls into place."

In the midst of her prayers and visualizations, Shirley says her phone rang. About fifteen minutes had passed since she had begun her prayer session. On the other end of the line was an assistant from the animal hospital.

"She said I could come over and pick up the cats because Sheba had quietly come out of her hiding place and could now be easily handled. She said the vet was incredulous that the situation was resolved so quickly."

For Shirley, the result was not all that surprising. "It was a very easy miracle." She laughs. "Animals will pick up from you exactly how you feel. I think we underestimate their intelligence. So if your cat—or any other animal—is in trouble, pray. I'm sure you'll see a positive effect, as I did."

25 · A Horse of Many Colors

ADRIEN Amadeo, director of the Internet-based Heal-apet Network, acknowledges that she was born with a special gift—the ability to communicate with animals. The Canadian-born healer and minister says she has always taken this unique talent for granted, although she remembers as a youngster never speaking too much about it for fear of public ridicule.

Today, however, as head of a popular healing network, the former schoolteacher is very much in the public eye and makes no effort to conceal her remarkable ability, which she often uses in her healing work with animals.

Adrien, who practices an ancient Tibetan form of energy healing known as Reiki, says that over the years she has undertaken many animal healings. But what she considers one of her most remarkable cases had to do with her own horse, Silver Morn. When the horse fell ill with a life-threatening infection, Adrien immediately sensed that more than veterinary care was needed. So she turned to a combination of prayer and Reiki energy.

The result of that spiritual healing can be seen by anyone who wishes to visit British Columbia. On a horse farm out there, Silver Morn can be found peacefully grazing, grateful for his owner's special healing touch.

• • •

Some people may think talking to animals is crazy. Not Adrien Amadeo, who recalls with a broad smile how, as a child, "I used to walk around and talk to different animals in my head.

"Birds would fly by and I just knew that they were talking to me. It was an intuitive feeling and it felt quite normal. It was only when I grew up that I realized this ability was something most people didn't accept."

The attractive blond-haired animal healer and communicator recalls that it was a gift that she could not share with her parents. "Although they both liked animals," she explains, "they were never lovers of animals, and I didn't think they would understand."

Adrian's father was an air-force officer, and the family moved around a lot. As a result of all this moving about, Adrien did not own a dog until she was out of the house and on her own at age eighteen. Since then, Adrien says she cannot remember a time when she hasn't owned a pet. "I've always had them around because I always had such a passion for them," she declares.

Her love of animals, along with her special gift of healing, is something the resident of British Columbia is convinced comes from a previous lifetime. "These kinds of strong feelings usually carry forth from lifetime to lifetime," she contends. "When you have a real passion for something, it's generally from a previous incarnation."

Although Adrien, who recently was ordained as a minister of healing by the Church of the Ancients, eventually decided to become a schoolteacher, she recalls always having an interest in healing and metaphysics. Over the years, she has studied everything from crystal healing and past-life regression to Reiki, an ancient Tibetan healing technique.

"I've always had a keen interest in alternative and complementary medicine, including acupuncture, herbs, and aromatherapy," she asserts. "But perhaps my biggest passion is animals—all animals. My love for the animal kingdom runs deep."

In 1998, Adrien decided to do something to help animals who were in need. As a Reiki master, she volunteered her skills with the recently formed Healapet Network, whose practitioners perform long-distance, or "remote," healings on ailing animals. Healapet was a dream come true for her. Now Adrien was able to combine her twin interests of healing and animals. Since taking on that work, Adrien has aided many ill animals, but one of her most dramatic successes involved her own horse, Silver Morn.

Her fondness for Silver Morn—whom she nicknamed Sugar—is evident whenever she speaks about her. "Sugar's a beautiful, gray part-Arabian who's twenty-seven years old and very healthy," she declares.

"I bought her when she was two as a pleasure horse to ride, then we got into things like Western riding and different competitions. We did a little bit of everything because she's an all-around horse."

Adrien recollects a summer day when she was routinely checking on Silver Morn, who had recently experienced some lameness in one leg. "I was rubbing my hands under her belly and I discovered a huge swelling. It was twice as long as my hands and hung down from her belly."

Adrien immediately called her veterinarian, who performed blood tests on the ailing horse. Vet Michael Perron told Adrien that Silver Morn had a serious infection, but he was not certain as to the exact source of the infection. He then went on to prescribe some antibiotics.

"That Friday we began the treatments," Adrien relates. "Michael cautioned that the edema wouldn't go away overnight. He said it usually takes weeks for the condition to clear up.

"The girls who worked in the barn agreed with him. They said they had seen this condition in horses they've cared for many times before, and it always took weeks before the antibiotics kicked in and the infection healed."

All of this did not sit well with Adrien. She fretted that the longer the infection lingered, the more danger it posed to Silver Morn, who was no longer a young colt. "I said to myself, 'We'll, see about that.' That day I began doing Reiki on her. I sent her healing energy. The next day, around eleven o'clock in the morning, I went to visit Silver Morn in her stall. The problem was still there."

Worried, Adrien then turned to prayer. "I generally pray to God for help when I do my healings, but this time I specifically asked that Silver Morn be healed *quickly*.

"I remember being alone in the barn with Sugar, and I was *really* praying hard. I had my eyes closed. There was no one else around, so I was able to focus. I said, 'God, please send Your loving healing through me so that I may help assist You in this healing of my horse.'"

In her conversation with God, Adrien explained just what was wrong with Silver Morn, including the antibiotics the horse was taking. "Then I started praying for God to send holy healing angels. I may not have gone to church much as a kid, but I was really focused. These were prayers from the deepest part of my soul."

After about ten minutes of constant prayer, Adrien opened her eyes. Checking the horse, she was again disappointed to find that the condition remained. She returned to her prayers, this time entering an even deeper meditative state. Soon remarkable images began to appear in her mind's eye.

"I saw colors that seemed to be directed at Silver Morn," she recalls. "There was a beautiful green color, and I saw spikes of white light shooting out of this green. I knew immediately that green was the color of healing.

"Then the color green all of a sudden turned to purple, which is another color that represents healing. When I envisioned these colors, I knew intuitively what it meant; healing was going on in response to my prayers. I just knew that I was witnessing a connection to the divine—a miracle."

The colorful display in her mind's eye was not quite finished. "All of a sudden that purple color turned to a beautiful silvery white. Silver Morn is a gray—almost white—horse, but this was a brighter color of white. It was silver white and it covered her whole body.

"When I saw that color, I knew without a doubt that she was healed and the infection was gone. I really can't describe it, but there was a feeling of peace and love that swept over me. I remember just standing there stunned—absolutely blown away by the whole experience. Then someone came into the barn, and it all stopped. I tried to get it back, but I couldn't."

Despite the dramatic mental visuals, the edema persisted. Had her visions been false ones? Two days later, she received an answer to that question. When Adrien returned to the horse farm to look in on Silver Morn, a surprise was in store for her.

"I looked at her belly and just couldn't believe it. The edema was all gone. You want to talk about a miracle—well, this was one of them."

Adrien remembers excitedly calling her veterinarian, who expressed doubt that the horse could heal so rapidly. "He just couldn't believe it," she recalls. "He gave the horse a thorough examination and could only shake his head in wonderment. The infection was, indeed, completely gone."

Reflecting back on that experience, Adrien submits, "You know, healings never surprise me. They just get me excited. I hope I never take any of these healings for granted. In this case, it was the power of prayer, along with the Reiki energy, that helped intensify the healing. It was also my strong desire to ask God for help. It was many things, all of them so intense that it was amazing."

And what did Silver Morn have to say about all this?
The animal communicator laughs at the question. "I
heard her 'tell me' she was feeling well—that the infection was gone. Then she put her head on my shoulder. I knew then that she was saying 'thank you.' "

26 . The Hard-Luck Chow

FROM the beginning, Chow Mein was a hard-luck dog. Abandoned and most likely abused, the two-year-old chow ended up at the Best Friends Animal Sanctuary in Kanab, Utah, where things didn't much improve.

While at Best Friends, Chow Mein was viciously attacked by the other canine boarders and nearly killed. When the shelter's veterinarian offered little hope for the dog's recovery, Amy Wagner, the adoption coordinator for dogs, refused to give up.

Amy, who admits to having a special soft spot in her heart for this unusual breed, extended not only prayer to the dying animal, but an extraordinary amount of love and care as well. The animal coordinator says she will never be quite certain what, exactly, caused the chow to beat the odds, but she's willing to bet on one thing—that prayer played an awfully big part in his miraculous recovery.

■ ■ ■

One of the reasons Amy Wagner gives for moving to
Utah from North Carolina, where she had recently
completed graduate school, was to find herself spiritually. "There was this whole spiritual aspect of me
that wasn't quite fully developed yet," the Pennsylvania native submits. "I needed to figure out who I was
spiritually, and I thought I could do so in this remote
state."

It was to prove a good move, because little did she
know that a seriously wounded chow who was under
her care would help her find what she was searching
for.

Amy says there was yet another reason why she relocated out west—this one a bit more practical. Although she had earned advanced degrees in English
literature and business, her dream was to someday
practice veterinary medicine. And what better creden-
tials to help her get into veterinary school than to work
at one of the nation's largest no-kill animal shelters?
Built in the 1980s, the Best Friends Animal Sanctuary
currently cares for more than 1,800 homeless animals.

"I grew up with an extreme love of animals—more
so than anyone in my family," she declares. "We always had cats and dogs around the house, and I was
always picking up strays and trying to find homes for
them. It was natural for me to dream about one day
being a veterinarian."

There was one problem with getting into veterinary
school, however. Without any science background,
Amy knew her chances of being accepted would be
difficult unless she, at least, had some field experience

working with animals. She had heard good things about the Best Friends Animal Sanctuary and decided to intern there. "I went out and liked it so much, I decided to go home, pack everything up, and return."

Since then, Amy says she has been kept busy doing what she likes the most—saving the lives of homeless and helpless animals. In the meantime, she is taking science courses to prepare for her future career as a veterinarian.

Turning to the story of Chow Mein, the adoption coordinator believes that her religious upbringing helped prepare her for her unique encounter with the chow. "I grew up in the Baptist faith, and I remember going to church every Wednesday and Sunday. There were always prayers said before meals, and bedtime prayers, so I'm no stranger to prayer."

When it comes to miracles, however, Amy says that although she grew up listening to stories of miraculous happenings in the Bible, she never expected to experience one herself. "This was a concept that I thought of as exceptional," she asserts. "It certainly wouldn't happen every day."

The miracle in her life began when a two-year-old abandoned stray by the name of Chow Mein turned up at the sanctuary. From the outset, the chow experienced difficulties. First he was not well accepted by the other canine guests.

"Chows are very aloof—very catlike in nature," Amy explains. "They'll come to you when they want attention. And unlike many other dogs, they're not pack animals; they're kind of loners. So they don't fit well into groups. They get beat up."

These attributes did not make for a warm welcome the summer day the red-colored chow with the black muzzle arrived at his temporary home, Amy recalls. "Once he was neutered and everything, he was placed into a group of other dogs that we thought would be a bit friendlier to him. We knew there were going to be some problems, but hopefully not serious ones.

"Chows not only have an arrogance about them, but they have this real fluffy fur and their tail curls around and sticks up. So in the mind of another dog, they look like they have their hackles up—like they're on the defensive—and this sends off bad vibes to other dogs."

For about a week, things seemed fine, and the staff at Best Friends thought everything would work out between Chow Mein and his new neighbors. They were wrong.

"We came in one morning and found that he had been viciously attacked—probably over and over again all night long. He was nearly gone. He was breathing, and that was about it. He wasn't responding at all. He had already gone into shock."

Amy and other staff members quickly swung into action. "We got some fluids into him, tried to feed him and get him up and moving," she recalls. "Nothing. There was still no response. He was dying." Although heartbroken, Amy was determined not to let this animal die. "So I carried him into my office to care for him, and I moved in with him."

In an extraordinary gesture of love and concern, for nearly a week Amy remained day and night in her office with the critically wounded Chow. "I would run home at lunchtime to take care of my own dogs," she recalls. "And at night I had somebody come by and

take care of them. I'd spend the entire night with Chow
Mein. I'd even sleep on the floor with him.

"Every day I would take him in my arms and carry
him out into the sun to see if he would perk up at all.
We tried any sort of remedy we could. We had him on
fluids, we had him on antibiotics, steroids, and we tried
any homeopathic remedies we could find."

Often, while alone with Chow Mein, Amy would
recall some of the religious lessons of her childhood—
something she had not done for many years. Prayers
she had uttered as a young girl while in church came
to mind, and Amy began to recite some of them. She
repeatedly asked God to spare this dog's life.

"I prayed for Chow Mein, but not on a daily basis,"
she says. "I also called somebody I knew in California
who loves chows, and she put Chow Mein on her animal prayer list.

"There were a lot of people praying for Chow
Mein's recovery—including our own prayer circle at
Best Friends. I even called my mother." She laughs.
"If anybody knows how to pray, she certainly does."

There was one day when Amy was informed by a
friend that she might not be reciting the right prayers
for the critically injured dog. "I was doing the prayers
that I would do as a five-year-old," she says. "I was
praying for things that I wanted—you know—'I want
this dog to live, please let this dog live.'

"Then, one morning, one of my coworkers, Joanne,
came into my office. She works in our 'Old Friends,'
department. It's a facility we operate that has about
fifty old dogs. She probably loses one of these old dogs
each week, and has learned to remain positive. She
said, 'You're not going to get anywhere in the

condition that you're in right now.' I was just crying all over this dog. I was sleep-deprived, I was food-deprived, I was not really fully functional.

"She also said, 'You're doing your prayers all wrong. You need not only to be sending out positive energy, but you also should be telling both God and Chow Mein that it's okay if the dog needs to go.' She told me I wasn't being fair in trying so hard to hold on to him.

"That switched my prayers around. Now I prayed, 'God, I'd like this dog to live, but if You need to take him, take him. I will understand that. Do what's best for the dog.' "

After almost a week, Chow Mein still failed to show any improvement. "He was now in renal failure. All his vital signs were off the chart, and his kidneys were about ready to go."

There was a morning, Amy recalls, when the shelter's veterinarian entered her office. "He took hold of my hand and walked me to the parking lot. He knew how attached I was to this dog, but said, 'Amy, things do not look good.' "

By now, Amy had become reconciled to the fact that Chow Mein would die. "I was now ready to let him go, but what really bothered me was that he was such a young dog. If he was fifteen years old, I would have more readily let him go," she explains, "but not at this young age when he was still at his best. He had been a happy guy, running around and enjoying himself.

"Then I asked the vet, 'Is he suffering?' He said, 'No, he's too out of it to be suffering at this point.' Despite the poor prognosis, Chow Mein managed to keep hanging on for a few more days."

Amy was full of despair, and one morning she entered her office, and had a heart-to-heart talk with Chow Mein. "I was feeling frustrated," she recalls, "and I said, 'Let me know what you want me to do, Chow Mein. If you want to go, it's okay.'

"I had to tell him it was okay for him to go, because I was afraid he was hanging on for my sake." She laughingly relates what happened next: "He just looked up at me and licked my face. I took that to mean, 'I'm still with you. I'm hanging in there.'"

Amy pauses a moment before continuing. "Whatever happened next, I think it was definitely the result of a miracle. This dog all of a sudden started to come around. It was a amazing.

"I think the miracle was a combination of things—prayer and the dog's perseverance—his will to live." What Amy modestly fails to add is the tremendous outpouring of love, prayer, and special care which she had given the chow for nearly a week.

To the amazement of virtually everyone at the shelter, Chow Mein was soon up and about. "No one could believe it," Amy declares. "About a week later, this dog who was on death's doorstep was up, moving around, and actually keeping his food down.

"The vet just couldn't understand what happened. All the blood work kept coming back that he was so far into renal failure, there was no way he could turn around from that."

Reflecting back on this episode, Amy says that the miracle she witnessed changed her life. "What happened with Chow Mein has certainly enhanced my spiritual life. I do think he came into my life and I came into his for a reason. All of this happened for a reason—and one of those reasons had to do with helping me to find myself spiritually."

The animal coordinator goes on to advise any pet owner who is caring for a critically ill pet never to lose faith. "Prayer can be a powerful tool for healing," she declares, "but don't be selfish with it. It's important to place the animal's fate in God's hands."

Amy adds that today, Chow Mein is no longer a hard-luck dog. "He is alive and well, living with his adopted family in Michigan," she explains. "He received a very special present this past Christmas when a Michigan family decided to adopt him.

"I took him there and I know that he's got a terrific home. I still hear all about him through E-mail and phone calls. He's doing just wonderfully."

▪ PRAYERS FOR THE ANIMALS ▪

1.

Heavenly Father,
Our human ties with our friends of
other species are a wonderful and special
gift from you;
We now ask You to grant our special
animal companions your Fatherly care
and healing power to take away any
suffering they have.

Give us, their human friends, new understanding
of our responsibility to these creatures of Yours.
They have trust in us as we have in You; our
souls and theirs are on this earth together to give
one another friendship, affection, and caring.

Take our petition for these, Your ill or suffering
animals.
Take our heartfelt prayers and fill them with healing
light

and strength to overcome whatever weakness of body
they may have.
Amen.

> *Anonymous*
> *Courtesy of Pet Prayer*
> *Line*

2.
Dear Heavenly Father,
In the same way as my little pets look to me, I also
come to you to ask you to meet our needs as only
you can.
Please help, guide, and protect all the little creatures
in the world.
Please save their lives, and give them food, shelter,
water, warmth, and good health.
Please be especially close to those who are lost,
abandoned, forgotten, neglected, mistreated, abused,
or exploited in any way and for any excuse.
Amen.

> *Anonymous*

3.
Heavenly Father,
Your goodness is turned upon every living thing;
Your Light flows from our souls to Yours and
touches each of us with the reflection of Your love.
To our special animal companions grant long and
healthy lives.
Give them good relationships with us, and if You see

fit to take them from us, help us to understand that
they are safe and peaceful in Your arms.
Amen.

*Prayer for Our Animal
Friends*

4.
Dear Lord,
Please hear our prayers for all the sick cats and
kittens.
Let them suffer no more and give peace to their
owners
so they can be comforted by Your will and have the
strength to face what may be in store for their
precious souls.
Amen.

Anonymous

5.
Good Saint Francis,
You loved all of God's creatures.
To you they were your brothers and sisters.
Help us to follow your example of treating
every living thing with kindness.
Saint Francis, patron saint of animals,
watch over my pet
and keep my companion safe and healthy.
Amen.

*Anonymous
Courtesy of Pet Prayer
Line*

6.

Hear our prayer, Lord, for all animals.
May they be well fed and well trained
and happy.
Protect them from hunger and fear and
suffering.
We pray, protect especially, dear Lord, the
little cat or little dog who is the companion
of our home.
Keep him or her safe.
Amen

Old Russian Prayer

7.

Dear Father,
Hear and bless Thy beasts and singing birds;
And guard with tenderness small things that have no
words.
Amen.

Anonymous

8.

Dear God,
Please let any little creatures who lose their life on
the roads, or any other place, be with You in Heaven
throughout eternity.
I cannot imagine Heaven without these innocent little
friends.
Amen.

Anonymous

9.

I lovingly share this planet with all of Creation.
I cannot imagine what life would be like without the
blessings of our animal friends.
I bless all of God's creatures in my prayers, knowing
that they, too,
are creations of the Lord.
Amen.

Anonymous

10.

Heavenly Father,
The bond we share with our friends of other species
is a wonderful and special gift from you.
We now ask You to grant our animal companions
Your fatherly care and healing power to take away
any suffering they have.
Give us, their human friends, new understanding
of our responsibilities to these creatures of Yours.
They have trust in us as we have trust in You.
Our souls and theirs are on this earth together
to give one another friendship, affection, and caring.
Take our heartfelt prayers for these, Your ill or
suffering animals, and fill them with healing Light
and strength to overcome whatever weakness
of body they have.
Amen.

Anonymous
Courtesy of Pet Prayer
Line

11.

May all that have life,
Be delivered from suffering

Lord Buddha

12.

May there be welfare to all beings,
May there be fullness and wellness to all people,
May all be full of happiness

Hindu Prayer,
The Upanishads

13.

How manifold are your works, O Lord!
In wisdom you have wrought them all—
The earth is full of your creatures;
They all look to you
To give them food in due time.
When you give it to them, they gather it;
When you open your hand, they are filled with good
things.

Psalm 104:24, 27–35

14.

Almighty God,
The animals are loving.
The animals are guiltless.
The animals respond to the
call and bring of life as we do.

To grow in spiritual understanding
Of these creatures,
To embrace them with warmth,
Makes me a responsible human being
Who can relate lovingly to all life.

Rabbi Joseph H.
Gelberman,
author of Zen Judaism

▪ CONTACTS AND RESOURCES ▪

E-mail Addresses

Adrien Amadeo, Healapet
Network .... adrien@healingspiral.com

Best Friends Animal
Sanctuary .... dogs@bestfriends.org

Carla Person, Shamanic
animal healer .... Carla@spirithealer.com

Dal Rescue .... DalRescue@egroups.com

Faithful Friends Animal-
Assisted Ministry .... Starbear@ghg.net

Melody Pugh, lost pet
detective .... Xoxonorman@aol.com

Pet Prayer Line .... PrayersForPets@aol.com

Prayer offerings for pets ... Petpray@gcstation.net

FORUMS

Best Friends: Prayers,
    Healing & Support_____ bbs@bestfriends.org

WEBSITES

Cat Chat _____	A message board for cat lovers.
Dalsavers.com_____	Very involved in dalmation rescue work.
Heartlight Message Boards _____	Prayers and much more.
Lightning Strike Pet-Loss Support Page_____	Many resources for getting pet owners through the hardest of times.
Melodykennels.com _____	Dalmation Rescue of Colorado.
Pet Pray_____	A prayer and support group.
The Woodro's Good Fight_____	Help in dealing with a pet's terminal illness.
World Animal Net Directory _____	More than 1,600 links to animal groups.

OTHER CONTACTS

Association for Research and Enlightenment _____	1-800-333-4499
Canine Companions_____	707-528-0830

Guide Dogs for the
  Blind_____ 415-499-4000
International Hearing
  Dogs_____ 303-287-3277
The Seeing Eye_____ 973-539-4425